SIE Exam Prep 2021-2022

SIE Study Guide with 300 Questions and Detailed Answer Explanations for the FINRA Securities Industry Essentials Exam (Includes 4 Full-Length Practice Tests)

Stephen Cress

Table of Contents

Introduction: The SIE Exam

Developed by FINRA, the Security Industry Essentials (SIE) Exam is an aptitude test that assesses the knowledge and skills of potential security experts. The test costs $60, comprises 75 MCQs (multiple choice questions), and lasts for 1 hour and 45 minutes.

The minimum age requirement to take the SIE exam is 18 years, irrespective of previous experience. The test scores remain valid for 4 years. Passing the SIE exam is one out of two important prerequisites to become a registered member in the security industry. Additionally, you must pass the qualification test for your prospective business.

The SIE consists of the following sections:

- Knowledge of Capital Markets — 12 questions; 16% of the exam

- Understanding Products and Their Risks — 33 questions; 44% of the exam

- Understanding Trading, Customer Accounts, and Prohibited Activities — 23 questions; 31% of the exam

- Overview of Regulatory Framework — 7 questions; 9% of the exam.

SIE Exam details

- Number of Items: 75

- Format: Multiple choice

- Duration: 105 minutes

- Passing Score: 70

- Cost: $60

- Recommended study time: 40 to 60 hours

You need a lot of studying and preparation under your belt to earn a passing score of 70.

Test-Taking Tips

Each time we are asked about how to pass the SIE exam, our response remains unchanged. Effective preparations for the SIE exam involve a combination of quality materials and an absolute commitment to studying. Though we are aware that each candidate is unique and there will be minor variations, there are a few tested and proven methods that are effective regardless of your study pattern.

We understand how overwhelming the SIE exam can be. For those who are looking to improve their performance during the test, this book is a helpful study tool.

If you have met someone who is exceptionally good at taking tests, you will understand how frustrating it can be. Especially when you have spent hours studying for the test, only for them to waltz through the process like it's nothing at all. This might be confusing. You might even begin to doubt yourself, asking how they could perform excellently when it comes to writing a test. How did they study? Which study materials did they use?

By now, you should be aware of the fact that performing well during tests requires skill. It is a strategic process where in-depth knowledge of the material is not exactly necessary. In simpler terms, it involves approaching the test strategically. In reality, there are similarities between most standard multiple-choice exams and there are a few, but effective pointers to "beat the test". The goal is to make sure that you become one of those individuals who pass the SIE exam with good scores.

Take it one at a time and pay attention to details. While this might seem straightforward, you will be surprised at the number of questions that people overlook because they hastily pick an answer without reading the question properly. It is an acquired reflex. We have been conditioned to read until we discover a tiny detail that points us towards the answer. We hold on to that tiny relevant detail and we just move with it.

This strategy is often effective and this is the reason why it is popularly used by many people. However, this method might prove to be the difference between passing and failing an exam, particularly one like the SIE. Hence, avoid self-sabotage. Attempt the questions carefully and scrutinize every word before selecting an answer. To ensure that there's no room for error, look through the questions again. With this, you can be sure that you understand the questions completely.

Rather than focusing on what you have no idea about, focus on what you know using the elimination method. The beauty of multiple-choice tests is that you have a chance to eliminate incorrect answers. For instance, if there are four options and you are sure that two options are incorrect, strike them out. This leaves you with 2 options and the odds are in your favour. If one out of the two options left is "all of the above", select that. It is most likely the correct option.

Alternatively, if after eliminating 2 options, you are left with one option that includes "none of the above", do not pick this option. Once more, statistics show that this is the wrong option. The correct answer is usually included by exam writers. Except you are absolutely certain that the correct option is not included, you should not assume that it's not listed

One other option to look out for when writing the SIE exam is "Not enough to determine". Once this option appears in the multiple-choice exam, do not select it. The information provided is ALWAYS sufficient. In reality, the information provided to answer the questions is more than enough. Regard this as a bonus option and strike it out immediately. This leaves you with 3 options to select from, increasing your odds of selecting the correct option.

Stick to Your Answer. Changing your answer leaves room for self-doubt. As long as you have carefully looked through the question before deploying the elimination method to select the most suitable answer, the odds are in your favour. Self-doubt eliminates all the logic from the method, reducing your final answer to a mere guess. What this means is that, when you change your answer, you are likely to select the wrong one, and this will reduce your scores. The most important thing to note here is to use the method and stick to your answer. There's a reason why you chose that option.

The Security Industry Essentials exam requires long periods of concentration. While it might be cumbersome, you must remain focused throughout. What this means that you should answer the questions you are absolutely certain about before going back to answer those that require more time. The only problem here is that it is impossible to skip questions during the SIE exam since the questions are generated by the computer and the preceding question must be answered before the next question is displayed. However, there's a way to bypass this hurdle.

Once you find out that a question requires additional time, pick any option. Then select "record and review", this allows you to continue the exam so you can return to that question later.

Preparation Tips for the SIE Exam

Without any doubt, the SIE exam requires effort. This is even made more difficult by the fact that you might be working full time when studying and you might have to write the test within a short period. By adopting effective study habits, you can maximize your chances of passing the test at the first try. Here are 15 tested and proven study habits for the SIE exam.

Dedicate quality reading hours. The SIE test is challenging and it requires many hours of reading. Set personal milestones, like completing a chapter, completing a test, and so on. Majority of the questions on the test will be new to you and anyone else writing the exam, so try to read every day because it is easy to forget important details.

Attempt and revise as many practice questions as possible. Getting information on the test is one thing, understanding how to answer the questions is another. I would recommend that once you equip yourself with all the necessary information, half of your study session will be spent studying the materials and the other half will be spent attempting practice questions.

Consider using sticky notes. Sticky notes can serve as effective bookmarkers in your study notes. Place sticky notes in the area of your note where more work needs to be done. Initially, your study note will be filled with sticky notes. As soon as you have grasped the information beside the sticky note, take it out and move on to the next one. Continue doing this, concentrate on studying the details beside the stick notes. Perhaps you might be able to complete the study sections next to the sticky notes before your exam.

Search for a quiet reading spot without distractions. If you want to increase your chances of passing the exam, you must remain focused. Stay away from the TV and even your mobile device or computer- except you are studying with it. Stay in a secluded area, you can stay in your car, visit the library, just make sure to stay somewhere you can concentrate.

Make sure to take a revision note or something similar everywhere you go. The importance of effective time management cannot be overstated. You might be presented with an opportunity to study for a little while. You can maximize this opportunity if your note or flashcards are with you.

Create personal flashcards. Create flashcards of the details you need to memorize. Take them with you everywhere so that you can look through them during your spare time. Once you have memorized all the details on one flashcard, set it aside from the rest.

Go on short breaks. There is a popular saying that people lose concentration after 20 minutes. Everyone is unique in their own way, and some people might be able to concentrate for an hour or more. Once you have gotten to the point where you forget a paragraph or sentence you just read, cut it out and go on a short break. A 10-minute break should help you to recharge, then you can continue studying after.

Read up on things you don't know. Avoid wasting valuable time by reading materials that you have fully grasped. Instead of this, focus on reading materials you are yet to understand.

Record your notes if you can. Several mobile apps can be used to make audio. If you are tired of looking through your book or reviewing test questions, take a few minutes to make audio recordings of yourself, read out your books. Then listen to the audio using your headphones whenever you have spare time or when you get tired of staring at your notes.

Understand the common terms. The SIE exam assesses your comprehension skills, this is why you must understand finance-related terms before taking the exam. By doing this, you will be able to understand the common terms used during the exam. When you are done, attempt the 75 practice questions. The questions in the SIE exam are curated by a committee, so you should expect variations in the question style. While one question has an interactive tone, another one might be filled with legal terms. Attempting the practice questions prepares you for these possibilities.

Multiple meanings might be attached to a single. It is worth noting that a single word might have several meanings. For instance, principal may be used to describe the manager of a brokerage company or the ability of a company on a particular trade, it can also be used to describe the face value of a bond. Furthermore, the word "covered" can be used to describe a protected position, it is also a popular term used when trading options.

A single concept can be described using multiple terms. In the same way one word might have several meanings, concepts can also be described using multiple terms. Terms such as shorting an option, selling an option, and option writing, can be used to describe the same concept. Once more, the test questions are curated by several individuals, so you cannot expect uniformity in the terminologies used, but the meaning of each term remains the same.

Although it isn't a math exam, three formulas worth memorizing. If you are in the security industry and math is one of the subjects you excel at, you won't be able to flex your mathematical skills in the SIE test. Most of the test questions are on reading and comprehension, there are only a few math questions. The three key formulas that you need for the exam are listed below.

- % load (sales charge) for a mutual fund purchase = (POP-NAV) / POP, where POP means Public Offering Price; NAV means Net Asset Value.

- Current yield = annual interest payment / bond price

- Dividend yield = annual dividend / stock price. Do not forget to multiply the quarterly dividend by 4.

Understand the application of concepts. One out of four questions in the FINRA SIE exam will assess your conceptual understanding. This is beyond having theoretical knowledge of the suitability of specific products. The test might assess your knowledge of the impact of Federal Reserve Board policy, and you can be required to find the relationship between three facts. For instance, you might be asked a question like: "If the FRB is hawkish, why do investors have to shorten their maturities?"

If you are taking the test, you must highlight the facts and indicate conceptual understanding. Hence, the following points must be highlighted in your answers:

1. The term "hawkish" is used to describe increasing rates

2. Due to the inverse relationship between price and yield, increasing rates results in a reduction in future bond prices

3. As a result of the reduced price volatility, the impact of rising rates on short-term bonds is lower in comparison to long-term bonds. Take note that the movement of the price is increased by maturity.

Another question might include customer characteristics such as job, risk tolerance age, and income. Then you will be required to estimate the suitable debt security recommendation. You must have a solid understanding of the safety profile and taxation value for each debt instrument. For instance, municipals are profitable for high earners as it is exempt from tax. On the other hand, investors who are opposed to taking risks might find treasuries more profitable since it is default-free.

Even if you are an exceptional test taker, taking the exam is quite challenging. The purpose of this book is to make things easier for you. If you can prepare diligently and use the tips in this book, then you can swing the odds in your favour. Once this book is used effectively, you can expect that it will be a step in the right direction towards passing the test.

Following the directions in this book, reading the materials diligently and preparing this test means that you are one step closer to a having fruitful career in financial services.

SIE Exam FAQs

When is the best time to register for the SIE?

While we recommend that your test date should be scheduled at the earliest possible date, nowadays it is easier to register for the SIE or other similar tests, than it was in the past. This is because the new exams are shorter.

How do I register for the SIE exam?

The exam date for the SIE exam can be scheduled directly with Prometric. Once you have registered for the exam on the FINRA website, you are required to schedule an appointment date with Prometric within 120 days.

What is the next step after passing the SIE?

Even if you pass the SIE exam, it does not automatically mean that you are qualified to operate in the security industry. Neither are you a registered member of FINRA by passing the exam. To become a fully registered member, you must pass a more complex exam like the Series 79 or the Series 6, which can only be written if you are associated with a licensed security company.

Do I get a second chance if I failed the SIE exam?

There is a 30-day waiting period after your first and second unsuccessful attempt. If your third attempt is unsuccessful, you have to wait for 6 months before retaking the exam.

What is the validity period of the SIE certificate?

The SIE certificate expires after 4 years. However, you are required to pass a top-off exam within that four-year period, otherwise, you might have to retake the test. Passing the top-off exam automatically means that you are a registered member and your SIE certificate retains its validity throughout the registration period, and for four more years after leaving from the security industry.

What is the recommended study duration for the SIE?

We recommend spending around 40 to 60 hours preparing for the SIE exam. This timeframe covers reading the materials and reviewing test questions.

What can I do to pass the SIE on my first attempt?

Every year, we prepare thousands of students for the SIE exam, and our goal has remained the same - 100% success rate. Follow our study guide, track your progress, and make sure your study plan is solid.

Chapter 1: Equity Securities

What is a Security?

In investment, security is a commodity that can be converted to a value, while taking chances. A security should be easily moved from one party to another, with the holder open to any loss of the initial capital.

Equity = Stock

Equity is also known as stock. There will be numerous words used in alternation for the purpose of this examination. Equity enables some sort of network between the owner or holder with the company involved. An investor becomes an owner of a firm when he buys stock in that firm. To set up capital, a firm trades its parts as shares to investors.

Equity securities are of two kinds: preferred stock and common stock. Preferred stock is not particularly preferred by every firm, but every publicly traded firm trades in common stock.

Common Stock

Many publicly traded firms trade in equity to raise working capital. Before any other kind of equity security is sold, every publicly traded firm must trade in common stock. Publicly traded firms have to take these steps illustrated below, for them to be able to sell their common stock;

Authorized Stock. This is the highest number of shares a publicly traded firm can sell to investors for fundraising purposes.

Issued Stock. This is a licensed and already sold stock.

Outstanding Stock. This is an already sold stock held by the public shareholders.

Treasury Stock. This is a stock already sold to the public, although these are bought back by the firm.

Values of Common Stock

Supply and demand decide the quoted price of common stock and doesn't necessarily indicate the real worth of the shares.

Book Value. The book value of a firm is determined by deducting all its liabilities from its actual assets. It is the value of that firm upon hypothetical liquidation.

Par Value. This is a means for the accountant to record credited money to the firm from prior stock sales.

Rights of Common Stockholders

Common stockholders have several rights in a firm because these investors are also owners of the firm. These rights are;

- Preemptive rights that ensures a stockholder can choose to retain their percentage interest in the firm. If the firm wanted to raise more principal, current shareholders must be offered new shares first.

- Common stockholders are joint owners of the firm, hence they own voters rights in the affairs of the firm.

- A stockholder's liability cannot exceed the amount of their principal investment in that firm.

- The majority of securities including common stock are easily transferred, hence, one can sell their shares with no need for authorization.

- Every stockholder has the right to audit the firm.

- If a firm is liquidated, common stockholders can get their equivalent interest in assets.

How Does Someone Become a Stockholder?

The majority of investors trade shares with other investors and this occurs in what is called "exchange" or "over-the-counter" market in the secondary market. Still, some investors buy from the firms when public offers are made. For a "regular-way" settlement, these are essential dates with respect to transactions;

Trade Date. This is when one's order is really effected.

Settlement Date. This is the day the equity buyer becomes owner on record.

Payment Date. This is the day when the equity buyer must have the money in the firm in order to purchase his order.

Violation

In the violation of Regulation T, the 4 business days permitted is exceeded without any payment by the buyer. Hence, the firm concerned can sell out the buyer's account or even freeze it.

Preferred stock

This has a fixed dividend rate which the firm is obligated to pay its shareholders. A preferred stockholder invests in the stock to get a fixed generated income via semiannual dividends.

Fractures of All Preferred Stock

Every type of preferred stock has similar fundamental features;

Par Value. This is what the dividend of preferred stock is established on. It is $100 until declared not.

Payment of Dividends. Preferred shareholders must be paid dividends before any common shareholders.

Thus, this gives priority claim to preferred shareholders.

Distribution of Assets. Preferred shareholders have priority claim on a firm's assets over common shareholders, in the event of liquidation or bankruptcy of the firm.

Perpetual. This explains why bonds have maturity dates and preferred stocks don't. Investors can hold their shares however long they choose

Nonvoting. At times, a cumulative preferred stockholder may get rights to vote if the firm doesn't pay as it should. However, this stock usually has no voting rights.

Interest Rate Sensitive. Preferred stocks have an inverse relationship with interest rate because it generates a fixed income. Hence, the higher the interest rates, the lower the value of preferred shares, and vice versa.

Types of Preferred Stock

Straight/Noncumulative. This type doesn't offer the owner any more than the basic features i.e. the fixed dividend rate.

Cumulative Preferred. If a firm cannot pay anymore, this stock protects the holder from that adversity.

Participating preferred. These owners hold rights to the basic features (fixed rate) plus common dividends.

Convertible Preferred. This type permits a preferred shareholder to convert their stocks to common stocks at the conversion price, which is fixed.

Callable Preferred. This type favors only the corporation. It enables the firm to call back in preferred stocks any time they wish.

Chapter 2: Dividends, Warrants, and ADRs

Types of Dividends

The economic status and the form itself determines what type of dividend is paid;

Cash. This is the typical way corporations pay dividends. It is done via checks. The brokerage firm pays in cash to investors directly using checks.

Stock. Investors who receive dividends in the form of stocks get extra shares according to how much they already had. This type is also used by the company to reward investors, and save cash.

Property/Product. This is not as common as the other types, although it's valid. Companies may choose to send parts of their property or products to shareholders.

Dividend Distribution

Dividends have to be paid to every common stakeholder. Outlined below is the process of dividend distribution;

Declaration Date. This is the day the company chooses to pay all its common stockholders. This is step 1 in the distribution process.

Ex-Dividend Date. This is the day from which shareholders no longer hold rights to receiving payment of dividends that have been declared to be paid.

Record Date. This is the day investors must ensure it's on record that their names are on the stock certificate otherwise they will hold no rights to receiving dividends.

Payment Date. This is the end of the distribution process when the corporation pays dividends to its shareholders.

Stock Price And The Ex-Dividend Date. It is essential to know that new buyers won't receive dividends already declared for payment, once the Ex-Dividend date arrives. This is because the price of stock before that date shows the price of stock with the dividend.

Warrants

This is a type of security that enables an investor to buy common stock. It comes at a subscription price that is more than the current market price of the common stock at the time the warrant is issued.

How Do People Get Warrants?

Units. If buyers buy the common stock of a corporation during what is called an initial public offering (IPO), the corporation will usually issue warrants to them. Units are common shares that come with a warrant to buy another common share.

Attached to bonds. Companies sometimes offer warrants as an incentive to bond offerings in order to appeal to the market. This enables the company to sell bonds at a reduced coupon rate.

Secondary Market. Warrants are as much in the market as common shares. Investors can choose to buy a firm's warrants instead of common shares.

Possible outcomes of a warrant. A warrant is similar to a right and an investor can exercise or even trade it. It can expire if the subscription price is more than the stock price on the expiry date.

American Depositary Receipts (ADRs)/American Depositary Shares (ADSs)

ADRs are receipts that show the ownership of shares held by a foreigner in a U.S bank branch. They aid the buying and selling of foreign securities in U.S markets. One ADR can stand for up to 10 shares of foreign stock and anyone with an ADR can ask for their foreign shares to be delivered to them. These receipts also make the holders entitled to voting rights and dividends declared for payment by the foreign company. If the holder's national currency depreciates with respect to the U.S dollar, they will get fewer U.S dollars as dividend payment and less when dividends are sold.

Functions of the Custodian Bank Issuing ADRS

On deposit, the custodian bank that holds the foreign securities can then issue ADRs. The bank certified as owner of the foreign shares must guarantee that those shares stay in the bank while the ADR remains unpaid.

Real Estate Investment Trusts / REITs

REIT is an unusual kind of equity security and is majorly for purchasing, advancing or managing a real estate portfolio. It is coordinated into a company and the publicly-traded REITs will trade on exchanges like other stocks and over-the-counter. A REIT won't pay taxes as a corporation if;

- Real estate is the source of 75% of its income.

- Nothing less than 90% of its taxable income is allocated to shareholders

Nontraded REITs

Any corporation that is involved in this business has to continuously ensure that the REITs are suitable before endorsing them. These trusts are more expensive, hard to value, and don't have liquidity. They can cost up to 15% of the price per share. Commissions and expenses are fees included and they have a limit of 10% of the offering price. However, this product appeals to investors because of the high yield presented. The similarity of Nontraded REITs to over-the-counter REITs is that they both have to allocate 90% of income to shareholders and both REITs have to submit reports to the SEC, annually (10-Ks) and quarterly (10-Qs).

Direct Participation Programs And Limited Partnerships

These are bodies that permit investors to gain access to earnings, charges, profits, losses, and tax gains. There are risks involved with no secondary markets for this business, hence, investors are advised to know the principles of these investments.

Limited Partnerships. This is a body that permits its partners to experience every economic occurrence, some of which include earnings, profits, losses, tax benefits, and decrements. This investment includes two kinds of partners, the limited partners and general partners.

The limited partners:

- raise principal for investment

- losses do not exceed their investment

- obtain extras from the investment

- can choose not to supervise the business

- have voting rights over the business objectives

- have voting rights over who is general partner

- can file suit against the general partner, if the latter acts to the disadvantage of the partnership.

The general partner can:

- trade in property for the business

- obtain settlement for supervising the business

- sign legally binding agreements for the business.

The general partner has to keep up an interest of nothing less than 1% in the partnership, financially. They CANNOT:

- merge their funds with that of the partnership

- contest against the business.

- be lent money from the business

At this level of business, one must understand that there are no consequences for tax. A DPP or LP has to keep away from at least two out of six characteristics of a firm if the partner wants to qualify for better tax treatment. These characteristics are;

- Continuous survival

- Purpose of gain

- Basic management

- Limited liability

- Colleagues

- Easily moved interest

Tax Deductions vs Tax Credits

Tax Credits cause a decrease in tax amount by the dollar expected from the investor. Tax deductions in partnerships are utilized in the reduction of investor's taxable earnings.

Chapter 3: Debt Instruments

Corporate Bonds

Bonds are issued by companies in order to start up their businesses. Corporate bondholders credit the company. They are neither owners of the firm nor do they have voter's rights. They can only vote if the corporation stops making payments promptly. The firm only pays interest on a loan till it matures, hence, corporate debt financing is also called leverage financing. If liquidation occurs, the company must pay bondholders before both the preferred and common stockholders. Investors receive generally taxable earnings.

Corporate Bond Pricing

Corporate bonds are valued at fractions of a percent as a percentage of par. For instance, if a corporate bond reads 95, its quote is:

95% × $1,000 = $950

A reading of 97.25 quotes:

97.25% × $1,000 = $972.50

Bond Yields

Nominal Yield. The nominal yield of a bond, also known as coupon rate, is invariably stated as percentage of par, and it is the "named" rate of interest imprinted on the bond. From the time the bond is issued, it becomes fixed. For instance, a holder with coupon rate of 8% will be paid an annual interest of $80.00.

8% × $1,000 = $80.

Current yield. This is the yearly interest produced by the bond with respect to its market price at present. It is calculated:

Annual income/current market price

Yield to Maturity. This is the entire annual earnings of the investor's investment in the bond.

Yield to Maturity: Premium Bond. An investor will have the least earnings if a bond is bought at a premium.

Yield to Maturity: Discount Bond. An investor will have the highest earnings from bonds bought at a discount.

Types of Corporate Bonds

Secured Bonds

This bond is reinforced by a particular promise of assets. These promised assets are taken as collateral for the loan. The title to the collateral is kept by a trustee, and the assets can only be reclaimed by the bondholders at default. Hence, the assets are sold off by the trustee in order to refund the bondholders.

Types;

- Mortgage bonds

- Equipment trust certificate

- Collateral trust certificate

- Bearer Bonds

Unsecured Bonds

These are called debentures, and they offer no collateral for the loan requested. It is supported by plain trust and reputation of the issuer. A debentures holder is like any regular creditor, in the case of default.

Types;

- Subordinated debentures

- Income/adjustment bonds

- Zero-coupon bonds

Guaranteed Bonds

For this bond, interest and main payments are backed by arbitrator like a parent company. The greater the reputation of the arbitrating company, the better the backing.

Convertible Bonds

This bond can be switched to common shares of the company at the conversion price which has already been fixed.

Convertible Bonds And Stock Splits

A company's declaration of stock Splits or stock dividends enables it to consequently modify its conversion price. While the bonds are unpaid, this bond's trust indenture declared the highest number of shares and minimum price at which they can be issued by the company.

The Trust Indenture Act Of 1939

Trust indentures are an agreement between a trustee and an issuer. They are issued when a corporation issues a surplus of unpaid $5,000,000 that was in excess of a year.

Bond Indenture

Bonds can be issued with a closed-end or open-end Indenture. A corporation that has an identical claim to the initial issue can issue extra bonds guaranteed by the same collateral if they are issued with an open-end indenture.

Ratings Considerations

The following factors of the financial condition of an issuer must be examined by a rating agency before rating any debt issue:

- Cash flow

- Kind of unpaid debt and the full amount

- Capacity to make interest and principal payments

- Collateral

- Economic flix and industry

- Management

The largest rating agencies are S&P and Moody's. An issuer can ask for and buy the service of either of these agencies if they want the debt of a corporation to be rated by one of them.

Exchange Traded Notes (ETNS)

ETNs are debt insecurities that establish maturity payment on the achievement of an index (an elementary security or group of securities). It is also called equity-linked notes or index-linked notes.

Euro and Yankee Bonds

Eurobonds are sold out of the country of the issuer, even though they are issued in the issuer's national currency. A Eurodollar bond is sold out of the U.S to investors although it is issued by a foreign investor in U.S dollars. Yankee bonds, on the other hand, are bonds in dollars that are issued by foreign issuers, and then sold to investors in the U.S.

Variable Rate Securities

Auction rate securities and variable rate demand obligations (VRDO)are the two major types. Auction rate securities pay interest at a rate that is readjusted at routine auctions every 7, 28, or 35 days. They are long-term securities that are sold as short-term securities. VRDOs pay interest at a rate that is readjusted at fixed daily, weekly or monthly intervals. A dealer fixes this interest rate to permit the pricing at part of the instruments.

Chapter 4: Municipal Bonds

The following can issue municipal securities:

- States

- Lands owned by the United States like Puerto Rico.

- Taxing authorities and their agencies made up of legal constituents

- Public authorities that manage mass transportation and ports.

Types of Municipal Bonds

- General Obligation Bond

- Revenue Bonds

- Industrial Development Bonds/Industrial Revenue Bonds

- Lease Rental Bonds

- Special Tax Bonds

- Special Assessment Bonds

- Double-barreled bonds

- Moral Obligation Bonds

- New Housing Authority/Public Housing Authority

Short-term Municipal Financing

All issuers including states and cities require short-term funding in order to supervise their available resources. They can sell their short-term notes and tax-exempt commercial paper. They sell short-term notes, expecting to obtain other income and then, Moody's service issues an MIG rating. These MIG ratings are on a scale of 1 (which is the highest) to 4 (the lowest). A state or city can issue different types of short-term notes like:

- Tax anticipation notes (TANs).

- Revenue anticipation notes (RANs).

- Bond anticipation notes (BANs).

- Tax and revenue anticipation notes (TRANs).

City tax-exempt commercial paper is typically supported by a credit line at a bank and its maturity date is

270 days (at maximum).

Government and Government Agency Issues

Series EE Bonds. Also called savings bonds, they are sold at a discount of about 50%, by the U.S government directly to the investors. They don't pay biannually and, they can be redeemed at stated value, when mature.

Series HH Bonds. Only investors trading in matured series EE bonds, can buy these bonds which mature after 10years. They are different from EE bonds in that they pay biannually and can be redeemed irrespective of maturity. They cannot be bought for cash, and they are available in sets of $500 to $1000.

Treasury Bills, Notes, And Bonds. These are the most common U.S government securities. The government is obliged to pay from 1month to 30years.

Treasury Notes. These intermediate-term securities mature between 1 year to 10 years. They pay biannually, and the treasury auctions them off monthly.

Treasury Bonds. These long-term securities mature between10 years to 30 years, and they pay biannually.

Treasury STRIPS (Separate Trading of Registered Interest and Principal Securities). Treasury STRIPS are bonds with zero-coupon which are supported by the U.S government securities. These securities are divided into two: principal, and biannual interest payment. An investor may buy a $1,000 principal part, set to mature in the future, at a discount.

Treasury Receipts. Unlike in Treasury STRIPS, banks and dealers generate these. They do this by buying huge sums of Treasury securities, putting them in a trust, and then selling the interest and principal payments to various investors.

Treasury Inflation Protected Securities (TIPS). TIPS gives investors security from the effects of inflation. They have a fixed interest rate, and their principal is reset twice a year to show the consumer price index shifts.

Agency Issues

These are particular organizations that have been licensed by the federation to issue debt securities.

Government National Mortgage Association (GNMA). This is a corporation fully owned by the government and it is also called Ginnie Mae. It is the sole agency that is completely grounded on the trust and reputation of the U.S government.

Federal National Mortgage Association (FNM). This is a for-profit public corporation, often called Fannie Mae. It involves public trading and its goal is to generate profit by supplying the capital.

Federal Home Loan Mortgage Corporation (FHLMC). This is also a for-profit public corporation that aims to make a profit on every loan. It is often called Freddie Mac, and it buys housing mortgages, then bundles them into pools before selling pool interests to investors.

Federal Farm Credit System. This is a group of private lenders who supply various kinds of funding to farmers. They provide with money gotten from sold farm credit securities. This is not supported by the U.S government and all the lenders on record are responsible for the securities.

Collateralized Mortgage Obligations (CMO)

A CMO is backed by mortgage and is issued by private financial firms, FHLMC, and FNMA. They have 'tranches', which are various set programs for maturity. They are set up like a pass-through deed. CMOs are collateralized by pools of mortgages on homes of one-family to four-family.

Types

- Principal only (PO)

- Interest only (IO)

- Planned amortization class (PAC)

- Targeted amortization class (TAC)

Money Market Instruments

These are readily available securities issued by firms of good reputation and are hence regarded as safe. They are fixed and have short-term maturity.

Corporate Money Market Instruments

To get short-term funding, companies and banks sell money market instruments, which include:

- Banker's acceptances

- Negotiable record of deposit

- Commercial paper

- Federal funds loans

- Repurchase deals

- Reverse repurchase deals

Government Money Market Instruments

- Treasury bills

- Treasury and agency securities with less than 12 months left

- Short-term discount notes issued by government firms.

Municipal Money Market Instruments

- Bond anticipation notes

- Tax anticipation notes

- Revenue anticipation notes

- Tax and revenue anticipation notes

- Tax-exempt commercial paper

International Money Market Instruments

Big organizations put their U.S dollars in foreign accounts for the greater interest rates. As explained before, these are termed eurodollars deposits.

Interest rate. This is the price of money. Both supply and demand for money, and inflation, determine the interest rate. Key interest rates include:

- Discount rate

- Federal funds rate

- Broker call loan rate

- Prime rate

- London interbank offered rate/LIBOR

Chapter 5: The Market Economics

Gross Domestic Product

The national GDP is a measure of the overall performance of the country's economy. It is best described as the value of all the products and services generated within the country such as investments, government spending, exports, and consumption during a specific year.

There is a constant fluctuation in a country's economy. Phases of increasing output are usually accompanied by phases of reducing output. There are four notable phases in this cycle:

Expansion. The expansionary stage is marked by a spike in the overall output and business activity. The economy expands or grows while there is an increase in wages, manufacturing output, savings, and corporate sales. Features of economic expansion include:

- Rising GDP

- Increasing consumer demand

- Bullish stock market

- Increased production

- Increased cost of real estate

Peak. Once the economy reaches a climax, the GDP hits the highest level for this phase while savings, manufacturing, and wages reach the highest point.

Contraction. The contractionary phase is marked by a fall in GDP, savings, productivity, and wages. The stock market plunges, unemployment rate increases, and inventories increase causing a reduction in business profits.

Trough. The trough phase sees a collapse in the economy as the GDP is at the lowest level. Savings and wages bottom out and unemployment peaks. The economy is ready to enter the phase of expansion to begin the cycle again.

Recession

The GDP declines during a period of recession, this continues for 6 months at least. The intensity and duration of a recession vary. During high-intensity recessions, the crash in prices affects the margins, pricing power, and profits of businesses. A reduction in consumer and business spending typically triggers a recession. During recession, there is a reduction in the overall demand since consumers and businesses pull back on spending.

Depression

During a period of depression, the GDP declines and this lasts for 18 months at least. The GDP falls by at least 10% during this period. The period of depression is the most intense type of recession and it is followed by significantly high unemployment rates and credit market freezes.

Economic Indicators

Leading indicators. These are the business conditions that change before a change in the economy becomes apparent. Leading indicators can be used to measure the economy's direction. They include:

1. Construction permits

2. Stock prices

3. Money supply (M2)

4. Fresh orders for durable goods

5. Average weekly initial jobless claims

6. Fluctuation in prices of raw material

7. Changes in consumer or corporate lending

8. Average weekly manufacturing work hours

9. Modified consumer goods inventories

Coincident indicators. Coincident indicators are reflective of changes in the economy. They are indicative of the current position of the economy. They include:

- GDP

- Industrial manufacturing

- Average personal income

- Employment rate

- Average number of hours worked

- Trade and manufacturing sales

- Nonagricultural employment

Lagging indicators. These indicators respond to a change in economic trends. Lagging indicators are used to validate the new economic trends. They include:

- Average duration of unemployment

- Corporate profits

- Cost of labour

- Levels of consumer debt

- Industrial and commercial borrowing

- Business borrowing

Schools of Economic Thought

There is a consensus among economists that low unemployment and minimal inflation indicate a thriving economy. Although each school of economic thought has its own beliefs on the effective approaches to restore or maintain a healthy economy.

Classical economics. Also referred to as supply-side economics, the classical economic model postulates that flexible government policies and reduced taxes increased employment rates which will result in increased demand and economic growth. Flexible business policies encourage the establishment of businesses and enable the production of goods at lower prices, creating more employment opportunities.

Keynesian economics. This economic model was first published during the Great Depression in 1936 by John Maynard Keynes. The theory postulates that healthy economic conditions can be achieved through a mixed economy achieved by the efforts of the public and private sector

The monetarists. The monetary economic theory postulates that economic trends and prices are influenced by money supply. Increasing the supply of money when there is high unemployment and reduced demand can help to improve the economy.

Economic Policy

The government attempts to controls economic trends using two instruments. The fiscal policy is regulated by the President and Congress and it affects government expenditure and taxes, while the national supply of money is determined by the monetary policy which is regulated by the Federal Reserve Board.

Tools of The Federal Reserve Board

The Fed attempts to control the economy by modifying the interest rates and the supply of money. The duties of the Federal Reserve board include:

- Adjusting the minimum reserves for member banks.

- Adjusting the discount rate

- Fixing federal funds rates.

- Sale and purchase of U.S. government securities via open-market operations.

- Modifying the amount of cash in circulation.

- Providing moral suasion.

Interest Rates

In simpler terms, interest rates refer to the cost of money. The demand and supply of money determine the overall interest rates, other determinants include the upward movement in the cost of products and services, or inflation. Other significant interest rates determine other rates.

The discount rate. This is the rate that the Fed charges on loans to member banks.

Federal funds rate. These are the rates that are charged for overnight loans among member banks.

Broker call loan rate. These are the interest rates charged by banks on broker loans used to finance margin trades.

Prime rate. This is the rate charged by banks on loans taken by their biggest and most reputable business clients.

Reserve Requirement

One way that the Fed can stimulate the economy is by reducing the reserve requirement for banks, this increases the lending capacity of the bank. Once additional money is provided to borrowers, there will be a reduction of the interest rates, resulting in a fall in the demand for products and services. However, this tool is hardly used.

Changing the Discount Rate

Another way that the Fed can stimulate the economy is by reducing the discount rate, this causes a reduction in other interest rates, reducing the cost of borrowing. Reduced interest rates promote borrowing and demand which then stimulates the economy. On the other hand, the Fed can slow down the economy by increasing the discount rate, this will increase other rates and increase the cost of money. The economy slows down once the cost of money rises.

Federal Open Market Committee

The Fed can stimulate the economy and reduce interest rates by purchasing government securities. This channels the money into the banking system and increases the amount of money that can be borrowed. The increased availability of money causes a fall in interest rates and an increase in borrowing and demand. The sale of government securities by the Fed slows down the economy. Once the money moves to the Fed from the bank, the supply of money is reduced. This reduces the amount of money that can be borrowed, increasing the interest rates and reducing demand and borrowing.

Fiscal Policy

This policy is regulated by the president and Congress and determines how the budget and government spending is managed. It might affect the level of taxation, federal spending, federal taxation, and the initiation or utilization of budget surpluses or deficits.

Under this policy, there is an assumption that the economy can be regulated by changing the level of taxation and government expenditure. An increase in government expenditure can stimulate the economy.

Numerous indicators are used by the government and the Federal Reserve Board to monitor the economy, they include:

- Price index

- Deflation/inflation

- Real gross domestic product

The stock market is significantly affected by both the fiscal policy and the monetary policy.

Yield Curve Analysis

The shape of the yield curve can be used by investors and economists to analyze the cost of borrowed money and the overall health of the economy. When the curve is normal, positive, or upward sloping, it indicates an increase in maturity which causes an increase in interest rates. When the demand for long-term loans is outweighed by the demand for short-term loans, the yield curve might be inverted, negative, or downward sloping, the curve also appears when the short-term rates are increased by the Federal Reserve Board to control an economy that is expanding too rapidly and may affect the long-term prove stability. An inverted yield curve indicates that the interest rates on short-term funds outweigh that of long-term funds. When the interest rates for long-term and short-term funds are almost the same, there is a flattening of the yield curve.

Fundamental Analysis

This assesses the financial ratios and financial statements of a company to determine the general financial performance of the company. The company's stock is determined by:

- Balance sheet

- Income statement

- Financial statement footnotes

- Accounting ratios

- Liquidity ratios

- Valuation ratios

Industry Fundamentals

Different industries are influenced by fundamental economic factors. The vulnerability of business earnings to a change in the economy can be determined by analysis. The 3 industry categories include:

Growth industries: In a growth industry, the company's earnings expand faster than the total growth of the economy. Tech and computers are growth industries.

Cyclical industries: Here, the company's earnings are extremely vulnerable to changes in the economy. The company thrives once the economy improves. Automobiles, raw materials, and manufacturing are cyclical industries.

Defensive industries: Here, the company's earnings are minimally vulnerable to any change in the economy. Production of military equipment is not under the defensive industry. Pharmaceuticals and food are defensive industries.

Chapter 6: Issuing and Offering Securities

Issuing and Offering Corporate Securities

The Securities Bill of 1933 was the first legislation used to regulate the securities industry, particularly the primary market. Transactions between investors and security institutions make up the primary market. During a transaction, the securities are sold and the funds are transferred to the issuer of the securities. The security issuer completes a document called the registration document, or the S-1. This document is reviewed by the SEC within 20 days at least. This is a time for "cooling-off" and no securities are sold during this period.

The Prospectus

While the registration statement is under review by the SEC, the activities of registered reps are limited. Registered securities are only permitted to receive indications of interest from customers by offering a red herring, or a Pre-IPO prospectus. Generally, the Pre-IPO prospectus includes a price list of the available securities. The details contained in a Pre-IPO prospectus are subject can be revised or altered.

The Final Prospectus

It is mandatory for the buyers of new issues to receive a final prospectus before any sales can be permitted. The final prospectus is the full-disclosure document issued by the seller to the buyer of the securities. Once the prospectus is being reviewed by the SEC and the final prospectus is available on the SEC website, a prospectus is said to have been provided to the buyer under the "access equals delivery" model.

Free Writing Prospectus

This is a form of written correspondence that contains the necessary information on the securities available for sale that falls short of the definition of a statutory prospectus. Popular examples include:

- Promotional materials

- Charts

- Term sheets

- E-mails

- Press releases

The Underwriting Syndicate and Exempt Transactions

Selling Group. A selling group is formed by a syndicate to promote issues. The members can only sell the shares to investors at a price called the selling concession, they cannot provide underwriting services.

Underwriter's Compensation. The underwriting syndicate comprises a group of brokers whose earnings depend on their respective duties. The lead underwriter is the only member that might earn the complete spread.

Review Of Underwriting Agreements By FINRA

Except for special circumstances, underwritten agreements must be submitted for review to the Corporate Finance Department of FINRA not exceeding 1 day after the registration is filed with the SEC or other state regulators.

Exempt Securities

Depending on the issuer or security, the 1993 Security Act does not apply to certain securities. Some of the exempt securities include:

- Debt securities sold in denominations of at least $50,000 or with less than 270-day maturity.

- Employee benefit plans

- Call and put options on indexes and stocks

Exempt issuers include:

- U.S. government

- Municipal and state governments

- Foreign national governments

- Canadian federal and municipal governments

- Insurance firms

- Trusts and financial institutions

- Credit unions and savings and loans

- Charity and religious bodies

Exempt Transactions

Occasionally, the type of transaction exempts security from the registration requirements under the 1933 Securities Act. Examples of exempt transactions include:

Private placements / regulation D offerings. This is the sale of securities to authorized representatives, the sales are exclusive and can only be accessed by authorized investors and people that:

- Are unmarried and earn a minimum of $200,000 annually

- Are married and earn $300,000 jointly, or

- Have a minimum net worth of $1,000,000 in the absence of primary residence.

The restriction on the amount that can be raised under the regulation D offerings include:

- $5 million under Regulation 504 D

- The unlimited amount under Regulation 506 D allows issuers to raise an unlimited amount of capital

Rule 144. The sale or restriction of securities is regulated under Rule 144. The owners of control securities include directors, officers, and stockholders with at least a 10% stake in the company. A private placement can be used to purchase restricted securities. Instead of a public sale, it can also be bought via an offering.

Restricted sticks can be resold to QIBs (qualified institutional buyers) under Rule 144. Any organization that owns investments worth $100 million or more is called a QIB. Examples include:

- Corporations

- Partnerships

- Insurance firms

- Investment firms

- Financial institutions

- Trusts

- Pension plans

- Authorized investment consultants

- Small business development companies

Regulation S offerings. Under the 1993 Securities Act, domestic issuers who distribute securities to offshore investors only are not required to file a registration statement for the securities to qualify for exemption under Regulation S, no offering of the securities must be made within the boundaries of the U.S. and the issuer must not publish or broadcast a written communication related to the securities in the U.S.

Regulation A offerings. The capital that can be raised under Regulation A was increased to $50 million under the 2012 JOBS Act. The exemption makes the capital market accessible to smaller firms without filing a full registration with the SEC.

Rule 145. Any reorganization or merger involving the company must be approved by stakeholders.

Rule 147 intrastate offering. This rule applies to offerings of securities that are restricted to a single state. To qualify for SEC exemption, the issue must have a principal business location and fulfill 1 or more of these requirements:

- 80% of the proceeds from the offering must be used in-state.

- 80% of the issuer's assets must be situated in-state.

- The majority of the issuer's employees must reside within the state.

Rule 415 shelf registration. Under Rule 415, issuers are permitted to register securities that might be sold for a subsidiary's benefit, its own benefit, or that is connected with business goals for a price that can be sold within 2 years by the issuer. This rule also permits the sale of securities continually, as long as it is related to the employee benefit plan or after other securities have been converted.

SEC Rule 405

This rule defines specific categories of issuers who might be allowed to use an exclusive registration process determined by the classification of the issuer. By filing the F-3 or S-3 form, experienced issuers can leverage the effective shelf registration of securities. Securities registered using Form f-3 or S-3 are effective immediately they are filed.

Issuing Municipal Securities

Choosing an Underwriter. Carrying out their duties and finding investors to clear the municipality's debt can be a daunting task for municipal officials. So, they usually assign a syndicate of underwriters or an underwriter to handle the bond sales.

Syndicate creation. A syndicate is formed by several investment banks, it helps with the promotion of the issue and to spread the risks of underwritten securities. A syndicate refers to a group of writers whose duty is to sell the issue.

Syndicate accounts. Each member of the syndicate must sell the bonds that have been assigned based on participation. There are 2 categories types of syndicate accounts: western accounts (or dividend accounts) and eastern accounts (or undivided accounts)

Submission of the syndicate bid. The terms and conditions of the bid can be set after a series of syndicate meetings.

Fixing the reoffering yield. The syndicate is tasked with allocating the reoffering yield offered to investors, the process is called writing the scale. Once the yield and prices have been determined, the bid and the necessary good faith deposit are submitted to the issuer

Awarding the issue. After the submission of all the bids, the bond council and the issuer must meet to decide on the syndicate that will be given the issue. The issue is generally won by the bid with the smallest NIC (net interest cost).

Compensating the underwriters. The spread refers to the difference in the price at which the bond is purchased by the underwriter and the price at which it is sold. The spread includes additional takedown, management fee, selling concession, and underwriting fee.

Order period. This is the time allocated for soliciting the bonds based on the order priority stated in the syndicate letter. It is done by the syndicate manager

Allocating municipal bonds. It is the duty of the syndicate manager to create a method for allocating bonds depending on the priority of orders. A written statement is required under the MSRB, and it is explained in the syndicate agreement, in addition to with the information regarding the sending of confirmations. The following orders might be received by the syndicate:

- Presale orders

- Group net or syndicate orders

- Designated orders

- Member orders

- Member-related orders

Sale date. Municipal bonds are exempted under the Securities Act of 1933, the cooling-off period does not apply to them. Hence, bonds can be sold immediately after the issue is awarded.

When issued confirmations. Once they have been awarded, municipal bonds can be sold almost immediately by the syndicate, even before they can be delivered physically. An initial or "when-issued" confirmation must be sent to investors who purchase municipal securities before the physical delivery.

Final confirmations. Once the certificate is available for physical delivery, the syndicate members are notified by the syndicate manager about the settlement date within 2 days, syndicate members must provide full payment of the bonds upon delivery. They are also required to send a final confirmation to the buyers of the municipal bonds before or upon the completion of the transaction, this is known as the settlement date.

Syndicate operation and settlement. After an agreement has been reached between the issuer and the syndicate manager, the syndicate manager must return the good faith deposits of other syndicate members within 2 working days.

The official statement. If the issuer decides to write a disclosure document, the issuer sends the official statement to investors. It includes all the necessary details on the issued bonds.

Bond counsel. The issuer is entitled to a legal counsel during the offering of municipal bonds.

Municipal Bond Trading

Like stocks, municipal bonds can be traded over the counter in the secondary market. Dealers share the quotes on their municipal bonds to other municipal bond dealers. The quote or two-sided market includes: (1) an offer, the selling price of the securities, (2) a bid, that is the price at which the dealer wants to buy the securities.

Chapter 7: Securities Trading

Types of Orders

The purchase or sale of securities can be executed using different types of orders. Once the order is not executed, all-day orders are canceled. A GTC or good till cancel can be used by the investor to keep the order active until it is canceled.

Market orders. This order ensures that the order is executed immediately it becomes available on the market

Buy limit orders. This order sets the highest price that the security can be purchased by the investor.

Sell limit orders. Investors use the sell limit order to fix the minimum price at which the security can be sold.

Stop orders/stop-loss orders. This type of order is used to guard profits and restrict losses.

Buy stop orders. This order is set higher than the market limit and it restricts losses or guards profits from the shorting of a stock.

Sell stop orders. This order is set below the market, it is guards against losses and protects profits from the purchase of a stock.

Stop-limit orders. The stop order and the stop-limit order are activated by investors for the same reasons. However, when the order is executed, it becomes a limit order rather than a market order.

Other Types of Orders

Investors can enter other types of orders that include:

- All or none (AON)

- Accept orders or Immediate or cancel (IOC) orders

- Fill or kill (FOK)

- Not held (NH)

- Market on close (MOC)/market on open (MOO)

The Exchanges

Globally, the NYSE (New York Stock Exchange) is the most popular stock exchange. Although several other U.S. exchanges operate similarly. Exchanges provide a central hub that connects buyers and sellers. The security listed on the exchange must be executed in the presence of an expert or the DMM (designated market maker).

The Role of Broker-Dealers and NASDAQ

Roles of the DMM as a principal. Once there are no public orders, the DMM must provide price improvement and liquidity for the stocks she's handling.

The DMM acting as an agent. Additionally, the DMM is obligated to execute the orders under her care.

Commission house broker. They are employed by a member organization, they are tasked with the execution of member's orders and the orders of member's clients

Two-dollar broker. When the commission house broker has too many orders to execute, some orders are executed by independent members known as two-dollar brokers.

Registered traders. Registered traders trade for their personal gain or loss. Registered traders trade actively on exchanges like AMEX, orders might not start from the NYSE.

Short Sales

If an investor thinks that a stock is overvalued and a decline in value is imminent, he/she can profit from this by shorting the stock. When shorting a stock, the trader borrows securities to complete delivery to the buyer.

Regulation of Short Sales / Regulation SHO

The SEC continually formulate new rules on the shorting of stocks. Regulation SHO is a modification of older short sale rules, it comprises:

- Definitions and order marking.

- Suspension of uptick rules and plus bid requirements.

- Borrowing and delivery requirements for securities.

Under Regulation SHO, SROs have been restricted by the Security Exchange Commission from fixing the price requirement before shorting a stock.

Rule 200 definitions and order marking. The definition of who can own stock is updated by Rule 200. Newer strategies, trading systems and derivatives have been formulated, amendments of the 1934 Security Exchange Act regarding short sales must be updated. Most of the old definitions and rules have not been changed.

Over the Counter/NASDAQ

NASDAQ is the National Association of Securities Dealers Automated Quotation System. Securities that are not listed on any of the popular exchanges are traded on NASDAQ or over the counter. NASDAQ offers a network of phone lines and computers that enable the trading of securities among brokers.

Market Makers

There are no experts for over the counter trades, so the offers and bids are communicated by brokers called market makers. Two-sided markets comprise of bids and offers quoted on the NASDAQ platform. Market makers are institutions that are obligated to show a two-sided market.

Broker vs. Dealer

Broker dealers describe the two roles that may be carried out by companies during the execution of a transaction. If a firm serves as a broker, it executes the customer's order at a commission. If the firm acts as a dealer, it partakes in the trade by acting as the opposing party. When making OTC trades, most brokerage firms usually act as the dealer.

Finra 5% Markup Policy

FINRA has formulated a policy to make sure that the cost of the securities is reasonable enough per market standards. FINRA regards a 5% charge as reasonable. This is a guideline, not a regulation. If a client's order is being executed at a low price, the firm might charge a minimum commission that exceeds 5%.

Chapter 8: Options

Options are categorized based on class, series, and types. There are two types of options:

Call options. With call options, a buyer is entitled to "call" or purchase a stock from the seller at a set price within a specified duration. Once the call option is sold, the seller is obligated to sell the stock to the buyer at the set price within the specified duration.

Put options. With put options, the buyer is entitled to "pull" or sell the stock to the seller at a set price within a specified duration. Once the put option is sold, the seller must purchase that stock from the buyer at the set price within the specified duration.

Bullish vs. Bearish

Bullish. Bullish investors are optimistic that there will be an increase in the price of a stock after a while. Investors who purchase call options are said to be bullish. This means that they expect an increase in the stock price and they have purchased the right to buy the stock at a set price referred to as the strike price or the exercise price.

Bearish. Bearish investors foresee a decline in stock prices. The stocks can be sold to the buyer at the set price since the seller expects a fall in the price of the stock.

Characteristics of All Options

The Options Clearing Corporation is the authority in charge of issuing and assessing the performance of all standardized option contracts. The American Stock Exchange and the Chicago Board Options Exchange are some of the exchanges where standardized options are traded. Each option contract represents one round lot (100 shares) of the underlying asset.

Managing an Option Position

An option trade is activated when the position is established by the buyer and seller with an opening transaction. The buyer establishes the opening purchase and the seller establishes an opening sale. Before exiting the option position, the position must be closed by the investor.

Buying calls. When a call is purchased by an investor, he foresees an increase in the price of the underlying stocks which would yield profits when the calls are bought.

Selling calls. When a call is sold by an investor, he foresees a fall in the price of the underlying stock and believed that he can profit from a crash in stock prices when the calls are sold.

Buying puts. When a put is purchased by an investor, he expects a crash in the underlying stock prices and expects to profit from the crash in stock prices by buying puts.

Selling puts. When a put is sold by an investor, he foresees an increase in stock prices and expects to profit from an increase in stock prices by selling puts.

Option premiums.

The cost of an option is called its premium. Options include out-of-the-money options, at-the-money options, and in-the-money options. These terms are not reflective of the profitability of the position, but they describe the relationship between the underlying stock and the option's exercise price.

Intrinsic Value and Time Value

The total premium of an option includes the time value and the intrinsic value. The intrinsic value of an option is the monetary value of the option. The time value is the price at which the premium surpasses the intrinsic value. This means that the time value is the price paid by an investor in order to access the option. Out-of-the-money options have no intrinsic value, so the total premium comprises of time value.

Using Options to Hedge a Position and Exercising Options

Long Stock Long Puts/Married Puts. An investor who holds a long position in a stock may protect his position from downside risk by buying a protective put

Long stock short calls/covered calls. Investors holding a long position can sell calls against the stock owned to get earn additional income and partial downside protection.

Short stock long calls. When a stock is sold by an investor, he/she expects to profit from a crash is stock prices by selling it at a high price and buying it cheaper.

Short stock short puts. Once an investor sells a stock short, he or she may be protected. To earn premium income, the investor can also sell puts against the short stock position.

Index Options

Indexes are instruments developed by experts for assessing the overall performance of the market. The most popular indexes are the S&P 500 (Standard and Poor's 500) and the DIA (Dow Jones Industrial Average). The two categories of indexes include; narrow indexes which monitor a specific industry, an example is the SOX (semiconductor index) and broad-based indexes which monitor a wide range of stocks, for example, the OEX (S&P 100) or SPX (S & P 500).

Index Option Positions

Index options can be used to establish the positions listed below:

- Long calls and puts

- Short calls and puts

- Long spreads and straddles

- Short spreads and straddles

- Long and short combinations

The Option Clearing Corporation

The Option Clearing Corporation (OCC) is owned and manages by the exchanges that permit options trading. The OCC issues and assesses the performance of all standardized options.

Investment Companies

Investment companies are either trusts or corporations. The fund contributed by each investor is collated in one account and the funds are used to buy securities that are most likely to help achieve the investment company's goals. A portfolio is created using the joint and each investor has equal stakes in the securities. An investment company assigns an expert to manage the funds of individual investors, these experts who only work with big corporations.

Types of Investment Companies

The Securities Act of 1993 regulates all the offerings of an investment company. Under this law, investment companies are obligated to register with the SEC and provide all investors with a prospectus. The Investment Company Act of 1990 also regulates the operations of investment companies. Under this Act, there are 3 categories of investment companies:

Face-amount company/face-amount certificates. An investor and a face-amount company can enter into a contract to receive a set amount of money at a specified date in future. The investor is required to make a fixed lump payment or pay in scheduled installments before he/she can receive.

Unit investment trust (UIT). Here, the investment is made either in a fixed portfolio of securities or a fixed portfolio of securities. A fixed UIT investment is made in a municipal debt or a sizeable block of government. The bonds are held till they mature and the profits are distributed to investors.

Management investment companies (mutual funds). Management investment companies employ investment managers to handle a diverse portfolio of securities created to attain their investment goals. These companies may be set up as closed-end companies or open-end companies.

Investment Company Registration

Investment companies must operate according to the stipulations of the Securities Act of 1933 and the Investment Company Act of 1940. To own, invest, or trade in securities, investment companies are obligated to register with the Security Exchange Commission. If the investment company has invested at least 40% of its assets in one of its subsidiaries or on securities that are not issued by the American government, then the company must register with the SEC.

Chapter 9: Mutual Fund Investment Objectives

Equity funds. The common stock is the only investment that will attain the company's growth target. Growth funds looking to increase their capital invested in the common stock of another company that is expanding faster compared to other corporations and faster than the economy in general.

Equity income fund. Here, both the preferred and common shares that have a longstanding history of consistently paying dividends are purchased. The fund buys the preferred shares at the stated dividend. Utilities typically pay the greatest percentage of earnings to stakeholders in the form of dividends, so utility stocks are also bought.

Sector funds. Mutual funds that commit at least 25% of their assets to a single industry are referred to as sector funds. Examples include gold, biotech, and tech funds. Sector funds typically have greater risk-reward ratios.

Index funds. Index funds have been developed to reflect the performance of a big market like the Dow Jones Industrial Average or the S&P 500. The portfolio of an index fund includes the stocks that make up the index that the fund has been developed to monitor.

Growth and income (combination fund). As the name implies, growth and income funds are invested to attain both current income and capital appreciation. One proportion of the fund's asset is invested in preferred and common shares that pay out high dividends, to generate income for the investors, while the other portion is invested in the shares of common stock with the highest potential for capital appreciation.

Balanced funds. This type of fund is invested in bonds and stocks using a standard formula. For instance, 30% of the fund's asset is invested may be invested in bonds and 70% in equities.

Asset allocation funds. This type of fund is invested in bonds, stocks, and money market instruments based on the projected performance of each market. For instance, if the fund manager believes that the stock market will perform well, he might invest more funds in the stock market. Alternatively, if he believes that equities will outperform the stock market, then he may channel more funds into equities.

Other Types of Funds

Bond funds. When an investor invests in bond funds, he is buying an equity security that corresponds with their undivided interest in a debt portfolio. The debt portfolio might have been issued by state municipalities, companies, or the American government.

Corporate bond funds. These type of funds are invested in debt securities issued by corporations. The debt portfolio might be speculative, as seen in a junk-bond fund or high-yield, or it might be investment grade. Taxes apply to the dividends generated by the interest returns of the portfolio.

Government bond funds. These funds are invested in debt securities issued by the American government including notes, bonds, and treasury bills. Some funds are also invested in the debt of government agencies, for instance, those issued by 'Ginnie Mae' or the Government National Mortgage Association.

Municipal bond funds. These funds are invested in portfolios of municipal debt. Municipal bond funds yield a dividend income, and federal taxes do not apply to them because the dividends depend on the interest payments generated from the municipal bonds in the portfolio.

Money market funds. Here, the funds are invested in short-term money market instruments that include commercial paper, banker's acceptances, or other debt securities that will mature within 1 year. With this type of no-load funds, the investor can expect maximally safeguarded principal together with the current income.

Valuing Mutual Fund Shares

The net asset value of the fund's shares must be estimated by mutual funds at least once every working day. The shares for most mutual funds are priced when the NYSE closes at 4:00 pm EST. The fund's prospectus offers the best solution on when the price of the fund's shares are calculated. This calculation is necessary to estimate the redemption price and the price at which the fund's shares are purchased. The price paid by the investor purchasing the shares and the price paid by the investor redeeming the shares are determined by the price which is estimated after the investor's order has been received by the fund. This is referred to as forward pricing. The fund's Net Assets Value is calculated using the formula below:

$NAV = assets - liabilities$

The NAV per share is estimated by dividing the total NAV by the total number of outstanding shares.

total net asset value / total no. of shares

Sales Charges

It is not permissible for an open-end fund to charge a sales charge more than 8.5% of the POP. The mutual fund's prospectus describes the sales charge that applies to specific funds. It is worth noting that the sales charge is the cost of distribution- which is the responsibility of the investor, it is not an expense of the fund. The commission paid to the underwriters, authorized reps and brokerage firms are deducted from the sales charges.

Front-end loads. This type of sales charge is paid by an investor after buying shares. The net asset value of the fund is added to the sales charge, and the shares are bought by the investor at the POP. Simply put, the sales charge is removed from the total amount invested, then the residual balance is invested in the portfolio at the net asset value. Front-end loads apply to unique shares referred to as "A" shares.

Back-end loads/contingent differed sales charge (CDSC). If an investment is made to a fund that charges back-end loans, the sales charge is paid when the investor redeems the fund shares. The sales charge depends on the value of shares to be redeemed. The longer the holding period of the shares, the lower the sales charge. The sales charges that apply to the back-end loans are described in the fund's prospectus. Back-end loans are charged by shares called "B" shares.

Other types of sales charges. Level-load funds are mutual fund shares that charge a level load determined by the NAV, they are also called "C" shares. Mutual fund shares which charge a back-end load and an asset-based charge are called "D" shares.

Breakpoint Schedule

Mutual funds reduce the sales charge depending on the amount of dollars spent, this is done in order to motivate investors to increase their investments in the mutual funds. These breakpoint sales charge reductions can be awarded to couples, trusts, corporations, and accounts for children younger than 18. Investment clubs, parents, or adult children with their own investment accounts are excluded from breakpoint sales charge reductions.

Breakpoint Sales

Should an authorized representative attempt to increase their commission by suggesting the purchase of mutual fund shares at a dollar amount lower than the breakpoint so that the investor can be awarded a breakpoint sales charge reduction, the representative is said to have violated the sales rule, and this is known as a breakpoint sale. This violation can also be committed if an authorized representative spreads out a substantial amount of money across several fund groups.

Rights of Accumulation

With rights of accumulation, investors can qualify for a reduced sales charge on future investments, after the value of the investor's account and its growth has been assessed. Contrary to a letter of intent, it is not time-bound, once there is a growth in the investor's account, the investor can qualify for a sales reduction on subsequent investments. This reduction does not apply to previous investments. The dollar equivalent of the present purchase is calculated into the total value of the investor's account before the investor can qualify for the breakpoint.

Automatic Reinvestment of Distributions

Investors can choose to reinvest their distributions into the fund and buy additional shares with the distributors. Investors can purchase most mutual fund shares at the NAV once the distributions are reinvested.

Closed-end funds. These funds are invested without a sales charge. To buy a closed-end fund, the investor must pay the current market price and the brokerage firm commission required for the order to be executed.

Exchange-traded funds (ETFS). ETFs have recently gained widespread popularity. They are formulated through the purchase of a pool of securities developed to monitor the performance of a sector or index. They do not require active management. Investors can sell, purchase, and sell short the ETFs at any time on a trading day. ETFs cost less and can be bought on margin.

ETFS that track alternatively weighted indices. One of the most common investment techniques is to invest in ETFs that monitor indices. For this reason, newer instruments such as fundamentally weighted, equally weighted, volatility weighted, and alternatively weighted ETFs have been developed to monitor the performance of alternative indices. They offer a fresh perspective on other investment techniques and often promise enhanced performance.

Chapter 10: Annuities

An insurance company and an individual enter into a contract known as an annuity. Once this is done, the individual is referred to the annuitant. There are three major categories of annuities, each with its own unique goal. The investment type and the means of investing the money depend on the annuity type. However, the ultimate goal of all three categories is to enable the tax-deferred growth of the investor's money.

Fixed annuity. Here, investors are offered a guaranteed rate of return irrespective of whether the guaranteed rate can be generated by the investment portfolio. Even if the portfolio performance falls below the guaranteed rate, the insurance company is still obligated to remit the payment.

Variable annuity. These annuities aim to increase the rate of return through mutual fund shares, stocks, and bond investments.

Combination annuity. Investors who think that the variable annuity is too risky and the fixed annuity is too safe can opt for a combination annuity, it combines the features of both variable and fixed. Combination annuities consist of a variable portion that aims to attain a higher return rate and a fixed portion that generates a guaranteed rate.

Retirement Plans

Individual retirement accounts (IRAs). An IRA can be established by any individual earning income. Tax may or may not be deducted from traditional IRA contributions, depending on the gross income level of the individual. Individuals who cannot partake in employer-sponsored plans can deduct their IRA contributions, irrespective of their income. There are four basic categories of IRA:

- Traditional

- Roth

- Simplified employee pension (SEP)

- Educational/Coverdell

529 plans. Otherwise called qualified tuition plans, 529 plans may be structured either as college savings or a prepaid tuition plan. The prepaid tuition plan allows the contributor to lock in the most recent tuition rate at their preferred school. It can either be structured as an installment plan or one where the plan is funded by a large deposit amount. 529 plans are guaranteed by many states, but contributors may be required to either be a resident of the state, or a beneficiary. Only tuition fees and other mandatory fees are covered by the plan. Some pans cover room and board options.

Local government investment pools (LGIPs). With LGIPs, local and state governments can manage their cash holdings while the current money market rates apply to the funds. If the yields of the offering are to be used to call in an unresolved bond issue, then LGIPs can be developed for investing the proceeds of that bond offering.

Achieving a Better Life Experience (ABLE) accounts. Also called 529 ABLE accounts, ABLE accounts are designed to serve as tax-efficient savings account aimed at helping people living with disabilities. Regulations guiding ABLE account were passed in recognition of the added financial expenses that come with caring for people living with disabilities. Beneficiaries can make tax-exempt withdrawals to cover current expenses incurred or to cover potential expenses,

Keogh plans (HR-10). This is a qualified retirement plan that can be used by sole proprietors, unincorporated entities, and self-employed persons. Corporations are excluded from Keogh plans. The plan can be funded with the income earned during the period when gross profit was generated by the business. Keogh contributions may be continued if the business suffers a loss. Participants must be vested by their employers after 5 years. Keogh funds can be withdrawn once the employee is 59.5% vested in their account.

Tax-Sheltered Annuities (TSAS) And Tax-Deferred Accounts (TDAS). These plans are set up as retirement plans for employees in public and nonprofit organizations.

Nonqualified corporate retirement plans.

These plans are funded with after-tax contributions, and the money can effectively grow tax-deferred. When a corporation contributes to the plan, the contribution may not be deducted from their corporate earnings until the employee receives their money. Distributions from nonqualified corporate retirement plans that are higher than the investors cost base, and they are taxed at the same rate as ordinary income. Every nonqualified plan must be written and the employer decides on the plan participants.

Qualified Plans

Every qualified corporate plan must be in written format and structured as trusts. A plan administrator or trustee is assigned on behalf of all the plan participants. Two main categories of qualified corporate plans include defined contribution plans and defined benefit plans.

Defined benefit plan. This plan is set up to provide participants with a defined/known retirement benefit plan.

Defined contribution plan. For defined contribution plans, the only known amount is the money deposited in the account, for instance, 8% of the employee's income. Money purchase plan, stock bonus plan, profit sharing, stock bonus plans, thrift plans, and 401K are examples of defined contribution plans

Chapter 11: Customers and Employee Conduct

Customer Accounts and Conduct

A salesperson must sign a filled form in order to start an account for a fresh client. There are 5 major kinds of account holding:

- Individual

- Joint

- Corporate

- Trust

- Partnership

Holding Securities

The stakeholder will then have to choose the system he'd rather have his bonds in, some of which are:

- Transfer and ship

- Transfer and hold in safekeeping

- Hold in street name

- Receipt vs. payment (rvp) / delivery vs. payment (dvp)

Types Of Accounts

Individual Account. An individual holds this account and he decides the transactions of securities within.

Joint Account. At least two persons can hold this account and both can make decisions concerning the account with or without seeking approval from the other.

Corporate Account. For a firm to have an account, the bank first ascertains the persons with the authority to decide on transactions for the firm.

Trust Account. This account can offer the benefactor of the trust (grantor or settlor) the right to nullify the account and retrieve everything they put into it. It can also be irreversible.

Partnership accounts. This account requires the bank hold a replica of a document stating which partner has the authority to make decisions on behalf of the firm.

Trading Authorization

There are other types of account that permits the occasional decision-making by a person other than was initially agreed. There must be a document licensing the elective authority;

- Discretionary account

- Custodial account

- Fiduciary account

Operating a discretionary account. This enables the banks spokesperson ascertain certain without having to ask the client;

- Which Assets to trade

- How much securities to trade

- Whether to trade at all.

Third-party and fiduciary accounts. A party other than the client supervises this account and determines the actions to be taken on behalf of the owner of the account. Fiduciaries are:

- Administrator

- Custodian

- Receiver

- Trustee

- Conservator

- Executors

- Guardian

- Sheriffs

Uniform gift to minors account (UGMA). Trading in securities is a deal bound by the law, hence the underaged cannot own an account without the supervision of the UGMA on behalf of the minor. These accounts require

- a custodian

- a minor

- the title of account stating the UGMA and State

- the account titled in the minor's name once they "become legal"

There are principles guiding the activities of the custodian to ensure they handle the account in the best interest of the minor.

Accounts for Employees of Other Broker Dealers

Numbered accounts. Some clients may hold accounts with numbers or symbols as the title. This is on the condition that there is a signed document proving them as the holder.

Option accounts. A client with the intent to buy or sell options, should have an option contract with the corporation and a replica of the disclosure contract.

Margin account. This basically enables a stockholder buy securities on credit.

Commingling Customer's pledged securities

This is not allowed unless both parties (clients) legally consent in writing to having their securities joined to the other's for the purpose of getting a loan.

Wrap Accounts

This offers guidance and administration to clients at a fixed yearly price. The account worth determines the price

Regulation S-P

This demands that the corporation follows certain measures satisfactorily, to ensure the information of it's clients are secure.

Identity Theft

Identity theft enables crooks to have illegal access to a person's financial information. Every bank and agent is obligated by the Federal Trade Commission (FTC) to develop and follow a written strategy to hinder identity theft. This requires an agent to include their strategy in their program manual. This strategy has to have warning signals and how to identify them based on common dubious patterns. This strategy must also offer the firm measures to effectively confront a case of identity theft and procure damage control.

Professional Conduct in The Securities Industry

Each agent has an obligation to supervise the activities of their stockholders as a result of the vastly controlled environment of the Securities industry. Every state has peculiar guidelines to be followed in the Securities industry, and failure to do so attracts a penalty and a dismissal.

Fair dealings with customers. As the heading implies, every agent must deal fairly and justly with clients by ensuring they adhere to 'rules of conduct' by FINRA. These rules supervise activities between agents and clients, and the manner in which they are carried out. They forbid:

- Churning
- Devious activities
- Illegal transactions
- Fallacious exploits
- Hidden suggestions
- Fabrications
- Excluding essentials
- Making promises
- Trading dividends
- Making suggestions on trading before verifying the client's risk taking abilities
- Temporary mutual funds business
- Exchanging fund groups

Mutual fund current yield. This yield refers to the annual dividends from a mutual funds and not the profits therein.

Disclosure of client information. It is illegal for a qualified spokesperson or agent to reveal information about a client to another person without their written approval or an injunction.

Borrowing and lending money. This is highly controlled and loans are only approved when strict protocols set by the corporation are followed.

Gift rule. A financial agent can only gift the client of another agent when the gift is:

- Worth less than $100/annum/person
- Received by the firm which then dispenses it to their clients
- Already accepted by the client beforehand

Outside employment. This is when a qualified spokesperson desires an outside employment with an associate company. They must first inform their employee who can choose to accept or decline.

Private securities transactions. A qualified spokesperson must obtain permission from the agent before making any private transactions. They must also have detailed records of everything concerning it.

Customer complaint. It is imperative that customer complaints be communicated as soon as possible to the director of the corporation.

Customer Recommendation and Taxation

NYSE/FINRA Know Your Customer (KYC)

All spokespersons are required to know the clients and their financial status well enough to be able to make appropriate suggestions that will suit the client's need. This KYC technique is important for the spokesperson to effectively do their job.

Investment Objectives

Stockholders have a common goal; to earn and secure their finances. This includes:

- Income
- Growth
- Preservation of capital
- Tax benefits
- Liquidity
- Speculation

Risk vs. Reward

Risk has a direct relationship with reward. It always yields some level of reward depending on how much risk is taken. Kinds of risks in investment include:

- Capital risk
- Market risk
- Nonsystematic risk
- Legislative risk
- Timing risk
- Credit risk
- Reinvestment risk
- Call risk

- Liquidity risk

Recommendations Through Social media

Social media posts are highly controlled by the corporation in question in order detect when information posts made by the firm becomes regarded as a suggestion or recommendation. This is very important for corporations as it is paramount that the suggestion suits the client's needs as stipulated in the FINRA rule 2111

Tax Structure

Progressive and regressive taxes are the two kinds of taxes. Progressive tax charges based on the amount of income earned. Examples;

- Income taxes

- Estate taxes

Regressive tax doesn't vary at all irrespective of the amount of income. Hence this is disadvantageous for those who don't earn as much as others. Examples:

- Sales taxes

- Property taxes

- Gasoline taxes

- Excise taxes

Investment Taxation

It is important that stockholders understand the effect of taxation on investment. Stockholders are likely to be taxed when they:

- Trade securities at a profit

- Trade securities at a loss

- Obtain a dividend income or interest

Taxation of interest income

When stockholders receive interest, they are likely to be taxed on it.

Gift Taxes

Gifts of $15,000/annum/person and below do not incur tax for the grantor, instead the tax is moved to the receiver's account. The reverse is the case for a gift of more than $15,000.

Withholding Tax

Agents are expected to hold back 31% of earnings from a trade or mutual funds if the stockholder hasn't proffered their tax ID number or social security number.

Alternative Minimum Tax (Amt)

Highly taxable things included in the taxable earnings of well paid people are:

- Interest on a few business revenue

- A few stock alternatives

- Increased devaluation

- Tax on investments that don't generate income

- Specific tax deductions passed through from DPPs

Chapter 12: Securities Industry Rules and Regulations

The Securities Exchange Act Of 1934

The 1929 market crash led to the enactment of the Securities Exchange Act in 1934. The secondary market is regulated by the 1934 Securities Exchange Act. Secondary market transactions include investor-to-investor transactions that are conducted in the OTC (over-the-counter) or exchange market. During secondary market transactions, the money is received by the selling security holder, rather than the issuing company. All businesses and individuals in the securities sector are regulated by the 1934 Securities Exchange Act. The components of the 1934 Securities Exchange Act include:

- Establishment of the SEC (Securities Exchange Commission)

- Mandatory registration of agents and broker dealers

- Regulation of the NASD (recently incorporated into the FINRA) and other exchanges

- Mandatory net capital for brokers

- Regulation of short sales

- Solicitation of proxies by public companies

- Mandatory separation of company and customer assets

- The Federal Reserve Board is authorized to govern credit extension for securities purchased under Regulation T.

- Regulating the supervision of customer accounts.

The issuers of publicly owned securities are regulated under the 1934 Securities Exchange Act. Issuers are also mandated to file 10-Qs (quarterly reports) and 10-Ks (annual reports) under this regulation.

The Securities And Exchange Commission (SEC)

The establishment of the SEC was one of the biggest accomplishments of the 1934 Securities Exchange Act. The SEC is a direct public agency and the highest authority in the securities industry. The Securities Exchange Commission is not a designated examining authority (DEA) or a self-regulatory organization (SRO) or a designated examining authority (DEA). As the name implies, self-regulatory organizations regulate their registered members, examples include the NASD (now part of FINRA) and the NYSE. A designated examining authority examines the records and books kept by a broker dealer, which can also include FINRA or the NYSE. Registration with the SEC is mandatory for all agents, securities, exchanges, and broker dealers. Exchanges are obligated to file a statement of registration comprising of the certificates of incorporation, constitution, and bylaws. The exchanges must relay every new regulation to the SEC. Issuers with assets worth more than $5 million and at least 500 shareholders are required to register with the SEC, file 10-Qs and 10-Ks, and conduct proxy solicitation. Broker dealers who trade publicly are required to register with the SEC while maintaining a set level of cash flow referred to as net capital. Broker dealers must send the financial statement to every of the firm's client. Furthermore, the fingerprint of every staff of the broker dealer who partakes in the sale of securities, who supervises other staff, or have access to securities and funds, must be stored in the firm's database.

Extension of Credit

Under the 1934 Securities Act, the Federal Reserve Board (FRB) is authorized to regulate credit extension by broker dealers for the acquisition of securities by their clients. Below is a list of the rules of the regulations of various lenders and the bill that authorized the regulation of their operations by the FRB:

- Regulation T: Broker dealers

- Regulation U: Banks

- Regulation G: Every other financial institution

The National Association of Securities Dealers (NASD)

The revision of the 1934 Securities Act created the Maloney Act of 1938 which enabled the establishment of the NASD. The NASD served as the self-regulatory organization for the over-the-counter market, and it was aimed at regulating the activities of broker dealers transacting in the OTC market. The NASD has been incorporated into FINRA and it has four primary bylaws which include:

- The rules of fair practice

- The uniform practice code

- The code of procedure

- The code of arbitration

The Rules of Fair Practice/Rules Of Conduct

The rules of conduct were formulated to guarantee the fairness and equity of public trades. Simply put, members must trade fairly with the public under this rule. The rules of conduct are also referred to as conduct rules or the rules of fair practice. The rules of conduct regulate activities including, but not limited to:

- Commissions and markups

- Retail and institutional communication

- Customer recommendations

- Representative claims

The Uniform Practice Code

This code stipulates a set of regulations that govern the transactions between FINRA members. The code regulates:

- Settlement dates.

- Ex-dividend dates.

- Requirements for good delivery.

- Confirmations.

- DK (Don't know) Payment procedures.

The Code of Procedure

The investigation of infarctions and complaints by FINRA is regulated under the code of procedure. This code governs the timing of the discovery of an unconfirmed violation of the conduct rules. This code does not involve money, it solely governs the violation of rules

The Code of Arbitration

This code offers an avenue for the resolution of conflicts. The code of arbitration offers a permanent solution to conflicts between a member and:

- Another member.

- An authorized agent.

- A bank.

- A client.

Becoming A Member Of Finra

Prospective members must meet FINRA's stringent conditions before the approval of their membership by FINRA. Companies that conduct interstate securities transaction with the public are mandated to register with FINRA. Furthermore, broker dealers must register with FINRA if they want to become a member of a selling group.

Registration of Agents and Continuing Education

Hiring New Employees

New employees are vetted and interviewed by the authorized principal of a company. The principal is tasked with investigating the applicant's personal and professional backgrounds. Except under special circumstances, new employees must be registered as associates of the firm. The process starts when the new employee completes and submits Form U4, also called Uniform Application for Security Industry Registration. This form is used to document the candidate's personal and professional information.

Disciplinary Actions Against A Registered Representative

If a recognized authority sanctions an agent, the situation must be reported to FINRA by the employee. FINRA must be notified if disciplinary action by these organizations:

- The SEC

- Exchange or association

- State regulators

- Clearing firms

- Commodity regulatory bodies

The following must also be disclosed to FINRA immediately:

- Allegations of forgery, theft, or exploitation of assets

- Guilty plea, conviction, indictment or no contest of a criminal case

- Should the firm become a defendant in a case higher than $25,000 or if the representative becomes a defendant in a case higher than $15,000

- A representative is facing disciplinary action from the employing firm or if the agent is charged to pay a fine higher than $2,500 or if agents are restricted from receiving commissions.

Resignation of a Registered Representative

If an authorized agent chooses to terminate their appointment with a member firm, Form U5, must be filled and submitted to FINRA within 30 days. An associate's registration cannot be transferred to another individual. The registration cannot be transferred across firms. The employing member firm is required to complete Form U5 and submit it to FINRA to finalize the termination of the agent's registration. The employing firm where the new employee is joining must fill and submit a Form U4 to start the registration process.

Continuing Education

Majority of the authorized principals and agents are required to register for compulsory continuing education programs. These programs are made up of a firm element and a regulatory element which are administered by broker dealers and regulators respectively.

Firm element. FINRA member firms are obligated to identify the inadequacies in the training of their covered agents and formulate a written training plan to make up for this deficit. This must be done at least once a year. Covered agents are authorized individuals who conduct the sale of securities to clients. The firm is required to formulate a plan that equips the covered employees with the prerequisite knowledge of the company's products. Additionally, the plan must include the potential risks and suitability obligations associated with the firm's investment products and strategies. Except if requested, the firm is under no obligation to file its continuing education program with FINRA. However, disciplinary action might be taken against firms that do not report their continuing education plan appropriately including the covered employee's adherence to the plan.

Regulatory element. For every registered agent who registered after July 1, 1988, their participation in the regulatory element is mandatory. They are required to participate in the computer-based training at an authorized centre two years after their first registration and subsequently after every 3 years. If an agent fails to meet this requirement within the stipulated period, their registration becomes invalid. Agents who have stopped practising for more than 2 years are obligated to take a requalification test and their regulatory requirement will be based on the date when the exam is passed for a second time or the reassociation date. Agents who stop practising temporarily, or for less than 24 months are not required to take the requalification test and their regulatory element is determined by their initial association date.

Chapter 13: Public Communications

Institutional and retail communication is used by member firms to maximize their brand awareness. There are stringent rules in place to certify whether communications with the public are done according to industry standards.

Regulation Best Interest

An amendment of the 1934 Securities Exchange Act led to the formulation of Reg BI (Regulation Best Interest) which was adopted by the SEC on June 5, 2019. Every agent, investment adviser, broker-dealer must uphold the rules of conduct that makes it mandatory for the firm and its employees to act in the client's best interest. Regulation Best Interest covers all the guidelines for the creation of accounts and account transactions. This means that the account must be created in the customer's best interest when suggesting that a customer registers for a TOD (transfer on death), fee-based or joint account.

FINRA Rule 2210 Communications with the Public

The regulations guiding member communication with the public was replaced by FINRA Rule 2210. Under this new regulation, there are 3 new categories of member communication, they include:

- **Retail communication.** This is described as a written communication sent to at least 25 retail investments within 30 days. The authorized principal must approve all retail communications before they are released. If FINRA discovers that a member is making false claims in its retail communication with the public, the member firm must file its retail communications with the public for the last 10 days with FINRA.

- **Institutional communications.** This is described as a written communication that can be accessed by institutional investors only. As long as the member firm has a policy on the use of institutional communication and the employees have been trained on how to use it effectively, institutional communication may be released even without the principal's approval. The filing requirements FINRA do not apply to institutional communication, similar to retail communication, institutional communications must be upheld for 3 years by a member firm.

- **Correspondence.** This describes written and digital communications between the member firm and at least 25 investors within 30 days. A sample of every correspondence may be reviewed using a set of guidelines put in place by the member firm. The member firm is also obligated to train their associates on the firm's guidelines regarding the correspondence and also document the training.

Securities Investor Protection Corporation Act Of 1970

The SIPC is a public agency that protects the clients if the broker-dealer fails. Broker-dealers who are registered with the SEC must also register with the SIPC, and they must contribute annually to the SIPC's insurance fund to make up for losses as a result of the incompetence of the broker-dealer. Broker-dealers who have defaulted in their payment cannot conduct any business until the payment is made.

The Securities Acts Amendments Of 1975

The 1975 Securities Acts Amendments of 1975 endorsed the MSRB (Municipal Securities Rule Making Board) to handle the regulation of municipal bond trading. There is no enforcement agency in the MSRB. For transactions involving securities firms, the regulations are enforced by FINRA. For transactions involving banks, it is enforced by the Comptroller of the Currency, the FDIC and the Federal Reserve.

Conduct of MSRB Members

The MSRB Rule G10 makes it mandatory for all broker dealers who are registered with the MSRB to send this information to their customers in writing:

- The broker dealer's registration with the MSRB and the SEC.

- The MSRM website address

- Details on the availability of the investment brochure and where the brochure can be found on the MSRB website

- Details on the measures in place to protect investors and the steps to file a complaint.

The Insider Trading & Securities Fraud Enforcement Act of 1988

The regulations guiding the use and disbursement of nonpublic material information are covered under the 1988 Insider Trading & Securities Fraud Enforcement Act. Any information that is solely available to insiders within the company is referred to as nonpublic information. Information regarding any situation which can impact the firm materially presently or at a later date is referred to as material information. Material information is exclusive to insiders as it is required for them to efficiently perform their duties. It is a criminal offence for an insider to use this information to profit from an impending change in stock prices. Any director, officer, 10% shareholder, or individual who has access to nonpublic material information, or their spouses are referred to as insiders.

Firewall

To advise the firm effectively, broker dealers who serve as investment bankers and underwriters must be privy to every information regarding the firm. Broker dealers must make sure that insider information is not passed between the investment banking and the retail trading divisions. These departments must be separated physically by the broker-dealer using a firewall. Broker-dealers are required to uphold written administrative guidelines to protect against unethical use or the spread of insider information.

Telemarketing Rules

Telemarketing calls are regulated by FINRA Rule 3230. During your exam, the telemarketing regulations may be listed as telemarketing guidelines, or under FINRA Rule 320 or the telephone Consumer Protection of 1921. Telemarketing calls aimed at convincing clients to purchase products, property, or services must be made in compliance with the stringent regulations. Under these rules, firms are required to:

- Restrict calls to the hours of 8 am and 9 pm, depending on the client's time zone.

- Have a do-not-call database. Persons on this list must not be called by any employee for 5 years.

- Provide the company's name, address, and telephone number. The caller ID must not be blocked.

- Formulate appropriate policies to uphold a valid do-not-call database.

- Formulate appropriate policies to ensure that the numbers called are not listed in the national do-not-call database.

- Train employees on calling procedures and how to use the do-not-call list.

- Include the company's name, address and telephone number in fax advertisements.

The Penny Stock Cold Call Rule

The enactment of the penny stock cold call rule was done to make inform investors of the risks associated with the purchase of penny stocks. Penny stocks are unlisted securities traded at less than $5 per share.

Violations and Complaints

The rules for investigating accusations of violations and complaints made against members or authorized representatives are stipulated in FINRA's code of procedure. These complaints are collated by FINRA member staff during their routine assessments. The allegations may also be made by clients of the firm or by another firm. If the complaint is made to the FINRA staff, FINRA still has to investigate the credibility of the complaint. FINRA starts the investigation by informing the firm or the associates about the complaint that was filed against them, the firm or associates will be required to send a written response. The requested information must be sent within 25 days after the request was made.

Resolution of Allegations

If FINRA discovers that the claim is unfounded, it may be disregarded without disciplinary action. However, if the claim is validated by FINRA, it can be addressed via a formal hearing or a summary procedure.

Minor Rule Violation

The MRV letter is typically deployed for minor violations. The highest fine is a censure and a $2,500 levy. The member firm or associate must accept the MRV plan, if offered, within 10 working days. Once the MRV letter is signed, the claim is neither affirmed nor denied, and the respondent waives the right to appeal the judgment. If the MRV plan is declined, a formal hearing is started by the Department of Enforcement to confirm the basis of the violation.

The Patriot Act

Under the Patriot Act (a sub-section of the Bank Secrecy), broker-dealers are obligated to formulate policies aimed at detecting questionable activities. Firms must appoint a principal to ensure appropriate employee training and strict adherence to the policies. Firms are required to develop a program to operate a customer database to confirm the client's identity.

FinCEN

FinCEN is a division of the U.S. Department of the Treasury. The objective of FinCEN is to secure the financial system, strengthen national security, and protect against fraudulent activities. FinCEN collates and controls information on financial operations, analyze and transfer that information to law enforcement agencies, and forge a global relationship with international agencies and similar agencies across other countries. FinCEN must routinely send an email containing a list of institutions and individuals to the appointed principal at weekly intervals. The principal is obligated to compare the list to the firm's client database. Once there is a match, the firm is obligated to inform FinCEN within 14 days.

Annual Compliance Review

A compliance assessment of every authorized representative, supervising locations, and OSJ must be conducted by the firm member at least once. Every 3 years, non-supervising branch locations must be reviewed directly.

The Uniform Securities Act

The Uniform Securities Act (USA) is a set of guidelines for U.S. states that is aimed at ensuring uniformity in the rules for each state. Also referred to as "The Act", the Uniform Securities Act determines the criteria for the securities administrator in each state. The state administrator is the highest level of authority on security matters in the state. The state administrator might be appointed or might be the state's attorney general. The state-specific regulations set by the Uniform Securities Act are called blue sky laws.

Investment Advisers Act Of 1940

The 1940 Investment Advisers Act regulates the activities of investment advisers who offer advice to customers for a fee. Under this law, investment advisers are restricted from revealing customer information to outsiders without the consent of the client, except if they are legally obligated to reveal the information

Tender Offers

Individuals or firms actively looking to purchase the outstanding securities of an issuing party in whole or in part at a set price must make a tender offer. Investors are only permitted to tender securities they own. Short tendering, or short selling a stock is not permissible.

Stockholders Owning 5% Of An Issuer's Equity Securities

Under the Securities Exchange Act, Form 13D must be filed by institutions or individuals who purchase at least 5% of the issuer's securities. Under Rule 13D, the purpose of the investment and the investor's portfolio must be disclosed to the SEC, issuing party, and the exchange.

Financial Exploitation of Seniors

Although many individuals lead active and productive lives even after they are 80, FINRA has formulated a series of regulations to safeguard the financial interests of persons older than 65. Authorized agents must understand the financial resources, requirements, and habits of their customers. This is particularly noteworthy for transactions involving seniors who may need the assets to cover specific needs and are more susceptible to fraud.

SIE PRACTICE TEST QUESTIONS

We have curated a few test questions to assess your knowledge and highlight the areas that you need to work on. Not to worry, we have also included the answers and a detailed explanation of all the questions. With this, you can also have a general idea of the questions to expect in the SIE test.

Take note that these questions are similar to the questions asked during the exam, but it might not be the same as the actual test questions. To prepare for the SIE exam effectively, you must be ready for questions on all sections of the FINRA SIE exam structure highlighted in the table above.

We have included the correct answers and explanations for the practice questions below. Attempt the questions without looking at the answers.

Mock Exam 1 - Questions

1. The Securities & Exchange Commission (SEC) was created by Congress in

    A. 1934

    B. 1933

    C. 1929

    D. 1940

2. The term 'disclaimer' is most often associated with

    A. The fact that unregistered securities are riskier than registered ones

    B. The fact that the government cannot guarantee the accuracy of the information in a prospectus

    C. The fact that no agent can guarantee a customer against loss

    D. None of the above

3. SIPC, the securities investor protection corporation is:

    A. An insurance entity that protects investors who are sold worthless securities

    B. A Congressional guarantee against losses in the securities markets

    C. An insurance entity that protects investors investments again market losses up to $500,000

    D. None of the above

4. In most cases, Federal Securities Laws:

   A. Are given the same weight as State securities laws

   B. Are subordinate to State securities laws

   C. Supersede State securities laws

   D. None of the above

5. Which of the following are not considered money market securities?

   A. ADRs

   B. T-bills

   C. Reverse Repos

   D. Commercial Paper

6. When a corporation goes public, it is issuing:

   A. Convertible bonds

   B. Preferred stock

   C. Common stock

   D. Any of the above

7. The term 'issuer' most often refers to:

   A. A corporation seeking to raise additional capital for expansion or modernization purposes

   B. A business that prints up securities certificates such as bonds and stocks

   C. A business that has satisfied the listing requirements of one or more approved stock exchanges

   D. A business, a municipality, or a federal governmental entity that is seeking to raise capital from the sale of securities.

8. Every publicly-traded corporation is required to have a transfer agent and a registrar. The primary distinction between the two is:

   A. The registrar keeps the record of all stock and bondholders

   B. The transfer agent ensures that dividend payments go out to all registered owners of record on the payable date.

C. The transfer agent transmits the payment for securities from the purchaser to the seller in all secondary market trades.

D. They are not different --- they perform the same function

9. One of the more attractive features of common stock is that:

    A. The stockholders have the right to choose Officers

    B. The stockholders have the right to vote on quarterly dividends

    C. One cannot lose more than one's investment

    D. Any of the above

10. When the market price of a company's common stock has reached triple digits ($100 or above), the Board of Directors may elect to declare which of the below to make the shares more affordable?

    A. A stock dividend

    B. Reverse stock split

    C. A stock split

    D. Any of the above

11. When a corporate Board announces a 10% stock dividend, shareholders know they will be receiving:

    A. money

    B. more shares

    C. neither of the above

    D. both of the above

12. Boards of Directors in the publicly-traded sphere are elected by corporate stockholders, using which of the following methods?

    A. regular voting

    B. cumulative voting

    C. statutory voting

    D. any of the above are possible voting procedures

13. Call option contracts are considered to have intrinsic value:

   A. when exercise price exceeds CMV

   B. when the option holder has exercised the option

   C. when CMV is equal to exercise price

   D. when CMV exceeds exercise price

14. Reinvestment risk is least present in:

   A. 4% 10-year AAA rated Corporate debenture

   B. Zero coupon Treasury Bond

   C. 2% 10-year Treasury Note

   D. 3% 10-year AA rated Municipal G.O.

15. All of the below are typical features of an ETF except:

   A. they often are sector-driven portfolios

   B. they are traded each day based upon 4:00 pm NAV

   C. they are marginable

   D. none of the above are exceptions

16. Accumulation units are most often associated with:

   A. ETFs

   B. mutual funds

   C. annuities

   D. life insurance

17. One of the most frequently issued money market instruments is commercial paper. Typically, this investment has a maximum maturity:

   A. of one year

   B. of 270 days

   C. of 180 days

   D. of 90 days

18. The Securities Industry Essentials examination gives a candidate

    A. the right to engage in phone solicitation of sales prospects

    B. the right to trade securities

    C. the right to take one or more of the top-off representative exams

    D. all of the above

19. Certain securities are marginable under Regulation T of the Securities & Exchange Act of 1934 except:

    A. NASDAQ stocks

    B. listed stocks

    C. options

    D. all of the above are marginal under Reg. T

20. When an investor is bearish on the broad stock market

    A. buying calls on the S&P 500 index is an appropriate strategy

    B. buying puts on the S&P 500 index is an appropriate strategy

    C. not investing in the market is an appropriate strategy

    D. buying mutual funds is an appropriate strategy

21. A customer wishes to liquidate 100 shares of ABC common at the market. If the current inside market is 904.78 – 905.57, the client's transaction will occur disregarding commissions and other charges at

    A. 905.57

    B. 904.78

    C. at a price agreed to between the firm and the customer

    D. at the last transaction price prior to entering this order

22. A market maker is obligated

    A. to maintain and honor firm quotes during trading hours

    B. to maintain subject quotes during trading hours

    C. to sell no less than one round lot to a customer inside the spread

    D. to buy no less than one round lot from a customer at its ask price

23. The spread between bid and offer

    A. is entirely up to the firm which is making a market in the stock

    B. gets wider as the volume increases

    C. gets narrower as the volume increases

    D. is generally fixed for the trading day

24. The so-called 5% policy pertains to

    A. mark ups, mark downs and commissions on retail secondary market trades in municipal bonds

    B. commissions on NYSE trades exclusively

    C. mark ups on retail OTC transactions excepting new issues

    D. none of the above

25. The principal difference between a selling syndicate and a selling group would be:

    A. commitment

    B. Eastern versus Western liability

    C. commissions earned

    D. all of the above

26. Stabilizing is a term generally used in Wall Street to refer to the practice of:

    A. price fixing of a new issue

    B. maintaining a market price at or near the POP of a new issue for the sole purpose of protecting the stock from decline during a new offering.

    C. preventing losses for investors who buy IPOs

    D. none of the above

27. Regulation SHO severely restricts short selling during the cooling offer period of a follow-on offering. Which of the below is true?

    A. shorting stock of a company undergoing a follow on offering is prohibited during the registration period.

    B. an investor cannot buy the new shares in a follow on deal if they have sold the outstanding shares of that issuer during the cooling off period.

C. an investor may buy the new issue shares on the offering so long as any short sale has been covered at least one business day prior to the effective date.

D. none of the above

28. The maximum coverage offered per separate customer under SIPC insurance was set by Congress at:

    A. $250,000 for cash and securities combined

    B. $500,000 for securities and cash combined

    C. $1,000,000 for securities and cash with no more than $250,000 for cash claims

    D. $500,000 for cash and securities coverage with no more than $250,000 for securities claims

29. Recommending a limited partnership DPP investment to a customer would be a defendable recommendation for a client:

    A. seeking flow-through tax benefits

    B. who is not risk averse

    C. who does not have an immediate need for liquidity

    D. any of the above

30. When growth is the principal objective of the investor, each of the below could be suitable except:

    A. defensive issues

    B. emerging industries

    C. growth mutual fund

    D. Technology ETF

31. Exercise of an equity put option involves the writer:

    A. selling the underlying instrument at the strike price

    B. buying the underlying instrument at the strike price

    C. selling the underlying instrument at the strike price less premium

    D. buying the underlying instrument at the strike price less premium

32. The hours of operation of the Chicago Board Options Exchange are:

    A. 9:30 am to 4:00 pm CT

B. 8:00 am to 8:00 pm ET

C. 8:30 am to 3:00 pm CT

D. 7:00 am to 7:00 pm CT

33. The primary difference between a stock dividend and a cash dividend is:

A. stock dividends provide the corporate shareholder with additional shares in lieu of cash.

B. cash dividends are tax-free if reinvested in additional shares

C. cash dividends are tax-deferred if reinvested in additional shares

D. stock dividends are taxable upon receipt

34. A customer complaint is formally defined as:

A. any communication from a customer or a legal representative of a customer regarding misconduct

B. any written communication from a customer or legal rep of a customer regarding an allegation of a violation of one or more securities rules or federal regulations

C. a written allegation of a violation submitted by a customer

D. none of the above

35. The least liquidity in the securities shown below would be found:

A. in securities traded on the Pink Quote system

B. in securities listed on regional stock exchanges

C. in T-bills

D. in general obligation issues

36. Among the reasons a corporate Board would declare a stock split

A. is to increase corporate net worth

B. is to decrease the annual dividend

C. is to reduce individual shareholders' percentage ownership

D. is to make the stock more affordable

37. Sweeteners as that term is used in the investment banking community refers to issue enhancements which include:

    A. warrants

    B. insurance

    C. convertibility

    D. any of the above

38. The Securities & Exchange Commission was formed as part of

    A. the Securities Act of 1933

    B. the Securities & Exchange Act of 1934

    C. the New Deal legislation

    D. none of the above

39. Which of the following investment instruments trades on an exchange at a market price not directly related to its net asset value?

    A. open end investment company

    B. private hedge fund

    C. put and call option contracts

    D. closed-end investment company

40. When a corporation announces that it is seeking additional equity capital through a sale of additional authorized but unissued shares,

    A. this is a secondary distribution

    B. this is a primary distribution

    C. this is an IPO

    D. this is a split offering

41. Among the differences between an introducing broker-dealer and a clearing carrying broker-dealer is that clearing firms:

    A. Maintain possession and control of securities and introducing firms do not.

    B. Are members of all major securities exchanges and introducing firms are not.

C. Are permitted to engage in investment banking and underwriting of new issues of securities and introducing firms are not.

D. All of these are differences.

42. Pre-emptive Rights and Stock Warrants have a number of similarities. Which of the below represent characteristics these products have in common?

I. Each has a fixed price at which the holder may purchase shares of the issuer's common stock.

II. The fixed exercise price for both products is initially set at a level below the current market value of the common stock.

III. These products are tradable on securities exchanges

IV. Both have relatively short-term expiration dates

    A. I, II, and III

    B. I and IV

    C. II and IV

    D. I and III

43. When reviewing the definitions of broker-dealers and investment advisers, one would find that:

    A. Broker-dealers can engage in securities transactions for compensation.

    B. Investment advisers engage in providing advice relating to the advisability of investing or not investing in securities for compensation

    C. An investment advisory firm must have an account at a broker-dealer in order to have the recommended transactions executed.

    D. All of these

44. Keynesian economic theory deals with:

    A. Controlling the economy through regulating money supply.

    B. Controlling the economy through budget/government spending and taxation policies

    C. Incentivizing responsible financial behaviors through Congressional legislation and agency regulations

    D. None of the above

45. A significant number of public investors do not have a solid understanding of how common stock is offered

to the public. Two methods are the secondary offering and the follow-on offering. Which of the below are true statements regarding these methods?

A. Secondary offerings involve the sale of new shares other than the first time a company is going public (IPO).

B. A follow-on is an offering of new shares other than the initial public offering (IPO).

C. Secondary and Follow-on are two different terms for the same investment banking activity.

D. Secondary offerings involve the resale of outstanding shares at market bid and ask pricing.

46. FINRA has promulgated various rules and procedures pertaining to the operation of broker-dealers and departments within member firms. The M&A Department:

A. Is tasked with supervising Managed accounts and Asset Allocation accounts.

B. Is in charge of rules governing the Member and Associated persons.

C. Creates the firm's procedures pertaining to Merger and Acquisition activity

D. Deals with Market making and inventory Acquisition for the firm.

47. Mitigation of the risk of loss in a bearish market can be achieved by customers with vulnerable long stock positions placing:

A. Sell limit orders

B. Buy stop orders

C. Sell stop orders

D. GTC orders

48. All investors with short option positions:

A. Have a contractual obligation to perform in accordance with the contract terms if the option is exercised.

B. Pay a premium in order to acquire the contractual rights associated with the option.

C. Must be considered suitable for short sales of stock in order to be permitted to engage in shorting options.

D. May close out the position by taking a long position in a corresponding option contract.

49. All of the following are full disclosure documents used in the sale of securities with the exception of:

A. Official Statement

B. Notice of Sale

C. Offering Circular

D. Prospectus

50. SIPC is an insurance organization designed to protect investors against loss:

    A. When their brokerage firm makes provably unsuitable recommendations

    B. When their brokerage firm fails to notify them of an impending stock market decline

    C. When their broker-dealer goes bankrupt

    D. When their brokerage firm loses or misplaces their securities.

51. Registered persons must complete the regulatory element of their continuing education within _____ of their second anniversary and every _____ years thereafter.

    A. 60 days; 2 years

    B. 90 days; 3 years

    C. 90 days; 2 years

    D. 120 days; 3 years

52. For a call option, the strike price is:

    A. The market value of the underlying security at which the option must be exercised

    B. The price at which the call holder can buy the underlying security from the call writer

    C. The breakeven point for the holder of the option

    D. The price at which the call writer must buy the underlying securities from the call holder

53. At withdrawal, pre-tax contributions and earnings in a traditional IRA are:

    A. Taxed at the investor's ordinary income rate

    B. Taxed at the investor's long-term capital gains rate

    C. Not taxed if the investor is at least 59½ years old

    D. Not taxed

54. A particular issuer of bonds chooses to engage a managing underwriter under a negotiated, firm-commitment underwriting contract. The underwriter chooses to sell the bonds using a selling group rather than a

syndicate. Who bears the financial risk of unsold bonds?

A. The managing underwriter

B. The institutional investors

C. The issuer

D. Selling group members

55. Which of the following pay interest on a semiannual basis?

A. STRIPS

B. Treasury bills

C. Treasury bonds

D. Treasury stock

56. What is the tax status of Keogh plans?

A. Non tax-deductible contributions and tax-free distributions

B. Non tax-deductible contributions and fully taxable distributions

C. Tax-deductible contributions and tax-free distributions

D. Tax-deductible contributions and fully taxable distributions

57. Which of the following is the best hedge against inflation?

A. Treasury bonds

B. Preferred stock

C. Common stock

D. Municipal bonds

58. What is the maximum maturity for commercial paper?

A. 30 days

B. 180 days

C. 270 days

D. 360 days

59. All of the following are true of the syndicate when bringing a new equity security to the market EXCEPT

A. They take some of the financial burden off of the lead underwriter.

B. They cannot back out of the underwriting agreement during the cooling off period.

C. The can sell their entire allotment of the new issue.

D. They are responsible for selling some of the securities to the public.

60. A broker-dealer just sold some stock out of its own inventory to a customer. The firm

A. Just acted as an agent in the transaction; and will make a commission.

B. Just violated FINRA rules and will be disciplined for the sale.

C. Just acted as a principal in the transaction; and may earn a markup.

D. Just participated in an OTC trade; and it occurred in the fifth market.

61. A shelf registration is best described as

A. When an issuer registers securities with the SEC and can sell them for a period of up to 3 years from the effective date based on market conditions.

B. When a US or non-US company wants to raise capital outside of the United States.

C. When a private company raises up to $50 million from both accredited and non-accredited investors.

D. When an issuer offers securities to up to a maximum of 35 unaccredited investors per year and allowed to raise an unlimited amount of capital.

62. How many consecutive quarters must GDP growth be negative in order for the US economy to be considered to be in recession?

A. 4

B. 3

C. 2

D. 1

63. A customer wants to exchange her US Dollars for Euros. What will determine how many Euros she receives for her Dollars?

A. The amount of euros received will depend on the equity market conditions on the major European exchanges such as the CAC & FTSE

B. The interest rate differential between the 2 central banks - the Federal Reserve and the ECB

C. The nearby euros futures contract

D. The spot forex exchange rate

64. Which of the following must be included in a final prospectus of a new issue?

A. The final offering price, The delivery date when the securities will be available, The underwriter's spread, The red herring

B. The final offering price, The delivery date when the securities will be available, The underwriter's spread

C. The final offering price & The delivery date when the securities will be available

D. The final offering price

65. What is a call option writer's risk?

A. Unlimited

B. Amount of premium plus strike price

C. Amount of premium received

D. Strike price minus premium received

66. Which of the following is issued by a GSE?

A. GNMAs

B. T-bills

C. Treasury STRIPS

D. CDSs

67. The amount that is paid for a call vertical spread is the difference between

A. The premium received for the long call and the strike price

B. The premium paid for the short call minus the strike price

C. The premium received for the long call and the premium paid for the short call

D. The premium paid for the long call and the premium received for the short call

68. Common stockholders do not have the right to vote on which of the following issues?

A. Stock splits.

B. Election of the board of directors.

C. Bankruptcy.

D. Issuance of additional common shares.

69. All qualified dividends for ordinary income earners are:

A. Tax-free income.

B. Taxed as ordinary income each year.

C. Taxed at a set rate of 15%.

D. Taxed as special interest-free income.

70. Your customer wants to invest in a conservative income-producing investment and is inquiring about GNMAs. She wants to know the minimum dollar amount required to purchase a pass-through certificate. You should tell her:

A. There is no minimum; you can invest almost any sum.

B. $10,000.

C. $5,000.

D. $1,000.

71. The state of Texas is seeking to raise $500 million through the sale of general obligation bonds. Which of the following will support the repayment of the bond issue?

A. Sales taxes.

B. Property taxes.

C. User fees.

D. Ad valorem taxes.

72. When making markets over the counter, the firm is acting in what capacity?

A. Neither.

B. Both.

C. Dealer.

D. Broker.

73. An investor is long 1000 shares of OnNet.com at $30 per share. To gain the maximum protection he should:

A. Buy 10 OnNet June 30 puts.

B. Sell 10 OnNet June 30 calls.

C. Buy 10 OnNet June 30 calls.

D. Sell 10 OnNet June 30 puts.

74. A mutual fund would be offered at a premium to its value if it's a:

A. Front-end load fund.

B. A nondiversified fund.

C. Back-end load fund.

D. No load fund.

75. Creating false activity in a security to attract new purchases is a fraudulent practice known as:

A. Front running.

B. Active concealment.

C. Painting the tape.

D. Trading ahead.

Mock Exam 2 - Questions

1. Investment company financial statements are sent to shareholders

    A. semiannually.

    B. annually.

    C. quarterly.

    D. monthly.

2. When a broker-dealer acts on an agency basis to help a customer complete trades, the firm normally is compensated through

    A. mark-ups.

    B. commissions.

    C. transaction surcharges.

    D. asset-based fees.

3. When opening a margin account, the agreement that customers sign to pledge their securities as collateral for a loan from the broker-dealer is the

    A. hypothecation agreement.

    B. loan agreement.

    C. re-hypothecation agreement.

    D. margin agreement.

    A. primarily connected to the strength of the underlying security.

4. A registered representative located in California makes a 7:30pm cold call to The credit quality of an exchange-traded note is

    B. always difficult to determine owing to the lack of disclosure required when selling these products to the public.

    C. usually very strong, since they are commonly sold by broker-dealers who must meet minimum capital standards.

    D. based on the credit worthiness of the issuer, typically the investment bank that structures the note.

5. a potential customer in New Jersey. This is

    A. permitted because the call occurred between the hours of 8am and 9pm.

    B. permitted as long as the registered rep had prior verbal consent from the potential customer.

    C. permitted as long as the potential customer is not on the do-not-call-list.

    D. prohibited because cold calls can only be made between 8am and 9pm in the potential customer's time zone.

6. When comparing rights and warrants, which of the following statements is TRUE?

    A. Rights are often added to bond issues as sweeteners; warrants are offered to existing shareholders to permit them to maintain their proportionate interest in the company when additional shares are issued

    B. Warrants have shorter expiration periods than rights

    C. Warrants protect shareholders against dilution, rights do not

    D. The exercise price of a right is generally below the price of the stock when the right is issued; the exercise price of the warrant is generally above the price of the stock when it is issued.

7. Helen opened a Roth IRA last year and wants to know what part of this year's contributions she can deduct. The answer is

    A. she can't deduct any amount.

    B. she can deduct 100%.

    C. it depends on her age.

    D. it depends on her income.

8. Investors whose bonds have been called as interest rates have fallen are now facing

    A. capital risk.

    B. reinvestment rate risk.

    C. inflation risk.

    D. credit risk.

9. Dollar limits on 529 plan contributions per beneficiary are set by

    A. the Municipal Securities Rulemaking Board.

B.   the federal government.

C.   the College Board.

D.   various states.

10. During the accumulation phase of a variable annuity, dividends, interest, and capital gains

A.   may be reinvested without any current tax liability.

B.   may be withdrawn with no tax implications.

C.   are taxed as capital gains if the contract is non-qualified.

D.   are taxed as ordinary income if the contract is non-qualified.

11. A customer requests in writing that his account statements be held by the firm while he spends the winter in Florida. In response to the customer's request, the firm is permitted to honor the request

A.   for a maximum of three months.

B.   for the time period specified by the customer.

C.   for a maximum of two months.

D.   for a maximum of one month.

12. With regard to the price of closed-end fund shares held by investors which of the following statements is TRUE?

A.   Shares are sold at a discount when the securities in the fund have increased in value relative to their NAV

B.   Shares are sold at the price calculated at the close of business on that day

C.   Shares may be sold at a discount or premium to their NAV

D.   The price is set by formula each business day

13. The order of liquidation in a limited partnership is

A.   general partner, secured bondholder, limited partner, unsecured bondholder.

B.   secured bondholder, unsecured bondholder, limited partner, general partner.

C.   secured bondholder, general partner, unsecured bondholder, limited partner.

D.   general partner, limited partner, unsecured bondholder, secured bondholder.

14. Which of the following is not an example of a restricted person under FINRA rules?

    A. The brother-in-law of a restricted person

    B. The child of a restricted person

    C. The uncle of a restricted person

    D. The spouse of a restricted person

15. Which of the following interest rates is established by the Federal Reserve Board?

    A. Money Market rate

    B. Discount rate

    C. Prime rate

    D. Fed Funds rate

16. All of the following sectors are considered cyclical EXCEPT

    A. hotel.

    B. furniture.

    C. steel.

    D. healthcare.

17. Which of the following events would subject an individual to a statutory disqualification?

    A. An indictment for a securities related felony 3 years ago

    B. A felony conviction 11 years ago

    C. A conviction for a securities related misdemeanor 9 years ago

    D. A conviction for a non-securities related misdemeanor six months ago

18. Pursuant to Regulation S-P, a broker-dealer must provide a privacy notice to a customer

    A. when a confirmation of a trade is sent.

    B. at the time a solicitation is made to purchase a security.

    C. prior to engaging in any securities business with that customer.

    D. when a statement of account is sent.

19. Which of the following regulators enforce the MSRB rules for securities firms?

    A.   Federal Reserve

    B.   FINRA

    C.   FDIC

    D.   Comptroller of the Currency

20. Noreen and her husband Jeff, residents of New York City, have just had their first child Ali. They are interested in opening a 529 Plan for Ali in order to save for her future college education. As a registered representative, it would be most appropriate to tell them

    A.   to invest in a New York state 529 as there may be certain tax advantages at the state level.

    B.   to invest in a New York state 529 as there may be certain tax advantages at the federal level.

    C.   it does not matter which state they open up a 529 Plan in as the distributions will be treated the same regardless.

    D.   to invest in a 529 Plan outside of New York state as there may be certain tax advantages at the federal level.

21. Trader R hears news from an underwriter that his firm will be buying a large block of XYZ Co stock. If R buys shares of the stock before the news is made public, he is engaged in

    A.   insider trading.

    B.   bid-rigging.

    C.   front-running.

    D.   rumoring.

22. A primary difference between Ginnie Mae and Fannie Mae/Freddie Mac is that Ginnie Mae

    A.   mortgages are only available for government subsidized housing, while the others are available for all real estate purchases.

    B.   only finances commercial mortgages, whereas the others finance home mortgages.

    C.   is a government agency that has the explicit backing of the US government, while the others do not.

    D.   is a publicly held company while the others are privately held.

23. If a customer wishes to open a short margin account and sell short 100 shares of stock at $15 per share, the customer must deposit

A. $2,000.

B. $1,500.

C. $1,000.

D. $750.

24. The theory that says the economy is best controlled through taxation and government spending is known as

  A. Monetarist economic theory.

  B. Classical economic theory.

  C. Keynesian economic theory.

  D. Open market operations.

25. Preferred stock includes which of the following features?

  I.Voting rights

  II.Priority over debentures in a corporate liquidation

  III.Dividends if declared by the Board of Directors

  A. I only

  B. III only

  C. II and III

  D. I, II and III

26. An investor sells short 100 shares of XYZ stock at 61 and buys 1 XYZ 65 call for 1.50 When the market price of ABC is 62. What is the investor's breakeven on the combined positions?

  A. 60.5

  B. 59.5

  C. 63.5

  D. 62.5

27. When opening a minor's account, the social security number to be used is that of the

  A. registered rep.

  B. custodian.

C. minor.

D. parent.

28. Which of the following organizations guarantees the performance of standardized options contracts?

A. CBOE

B. OCC

C. SEC

D. FINRA

29. In order to receive a dividend, a shareholder must own stock as of the

A. ex-dividend date.

B. declaration date.

C. payable date.

D. record date.

30. A municipal finance professional at JoeBrokerDealer made a contribution of $500 to candidate in a local election that resulted in a ban on underwriting activity. A month later the MFP joined a new municipal securities firm, JaneBrokerDealer. The remainder of the two-year ban will apply to

A. both JoeBrokerDealer and JaneBrokerDealer.

B. neither JoeBrokerDealer or JaneBrokerDealer.

C. JaneBrokerDealer only.

D. JoeBrokerDealer only.

31. A representative's personal account has been identified for review because of account activity in which securities were bought and quickly sold, often on the following day. This may be evidence of the prohibited practice called

A. front-running.

B. selling away.

C. commingling.

D. freeriding.

32. When calculating total return on a bond,

A. interest earned is subtracted from any capital gain, and this result is then divided by the initial purchase price.

B. interest earned is subtracted from the redemption value of the bond.

C. interest earned is added to any capital gain, and this result is then divided by the initial purchase price.

D. interest earned is divided by the redemption value of the bond.

33. A communication made available to 20 institutional clients and 20 retail clients is classified as

A. institutional communication.

B. retail communication.

C. a blog post.

D. correspondence.

34. All the following are exempt from the registration requirements of the Securities Act of 1933 except

A. domestic bank securities.

B. US Treasury bonds.

C. AAA rated corporate bonds.

D. A rated municipal bonds.

35. The threshold to qualify for a sales charge discount on a mutual fund is $75,000. An investor places an order for $72,500 of this fund and is not informed by the registered rep that he would be entitled to a sales charge discount if he invests an additional $2,500. This is an example of a

A. letter of intent.

B. breakpoint.

C. value investor.

D. breakpoint sale.

36. Bonds that are issued by state and local governments but benefit a private corporate are

A. industrial revenue bonds.

B. double-barreled bonds.

C. moral obligation bonds.

D. special assessment bonds.

37. An upward sloping yield curve indicates

    A. that yields are falling.

    B. that bond prices are increasing.

    C. the Federal Reserve Board is pursuing a tight monetary policy.

    D. that long-term interest rates are higher that short-term interest rates.

38. Accrued interest is calculated from the

    A. last coupon date and continues to the day prior to the settlement date.

    B. dated date and continues to the settlement date.

    C. dated date to the next coupon date.

    D. last coupon date and continues through the settlement date.

39. Which of the following terms describes a broker-dealer's practice of interjecting another broker-dealer into the middle of a trade, resulting in an increase in commission at the customer's expense?

    A. Churning

    B. Front-running

    C. Collaboration

    D. Interpositioning

40. Penny stocks present added risk to customers because of

    A. their high surrender charges.

    B. their potential lack of liquidity.

    C. their potential for exposure to adverse tax consequences.

    D. their low potential for return.

41. For existing customer accounts, how often do broker-dealers required to send a written notice to the customer for verification of account information?

    A. Every 5 years

    B. Every 3 years

C. Every two years

D. Annually

42. Commercial paper, bankers' acceptances and large time deposits are part of what segment of the fixed income market?

A. Money market

B. Asset-backed

C. Municipal

D. Corporate bonds

43. Joe is a registered rep currently employed by MidWest Broker-Dealer, a St. Louis based firm. Joe likes to leave downtown and drive through the rural fields of the Midwest on the weekends. He so enjoys the open plains that he chats with his 12 closest family members to borrow $200,000 and open his very own farm. Which of the following is true regarding this action?

A. Joe must notify MidWest that he is engaging in outside business activity

B. Joe must notify MidWest that he is borrowing money from family members

C. This type of outside business activity is prohibited by FINRA rules

D. Joe must notify MidWest that he is engaging in an outside business activity and must await permission from his firm before moving forward

44. A company "reverse splits" its stock on a 1-for-10 basis. If an investor holds 800 shares before the event, what will be the impact of the split, if any, on the total value of the investors' shares?

A. Total value will decline by 90%

B. Total value will decline by 10%

C. Total value will not change

D. Total value will increase by 10 times

45. Which of the bonds listed below would have the greatest price volatility?

A. A long-term zero-coupon bond

B. A short-term investment grade bond

C. A Treasury note

D.   A variable rate bond

46. A corporate bond that is currently trading at 95 pays a semi-annual coupon of $25. What is the current yield?

   A.   0.0526

   B.   0.05

   C.   0.0263

   D.   0.025

47. Investors purchase common stock primarily for

   A.   its appreciation potential.

   B.   its resistance to business risk.

   C.   the income stream it generates.

   D.   its relative safety.

48. The Nasdaq market is a(n)

   A.   auction market.

   B.   negotiated market.

   C.   double-auction market.

   D.   transfer market.

49. To avoid double taxation on dividends paid to shareholders, REITs must invest what portion of their total assets in real estate?

   A.   At least 51%

   B.   At least 75%

   C.   At least 90%

   D.   Substantially all

50. A customer deposits $2,000 of cash into a brokerage account in the morning and $10,000 in cash into the same account that afternoon. The firm is required to file

   A.   a CMIR.

   B.   a CTR.

C. a SAR.

D. nothing at this time, but this suspicious activity should be monitored.

51. A husband and wife wish to open a brokerage account in which the husband will own 60% and the wife 40%. At either owner's death, the owner's portion will be liquidated and distributed to his/her beneficiary. What type of account should they open?

A. Tenancy by the Entirety

B. Joint Tenancy with Rights of Survivorship

C. Tenancy in common

D. Partnership

52. As part of Rule 144A, the SEC created another category of financially sophisticated investors known as

A. sophisticated wealthy individuals.

B. accredited investors.

C. qualified asset managers.

D. qualified institutional buyers.

53. What tax benefit do municipal bonds offer to individual U.S. investors?

A. Investment tax credits

B. Low tax rates on capital gains

C. Avoidance of Alternative Minimum Tax

D. Tax-exempt interest

54. When the market price of a bond is lower than its par value,

A. its current yield is lower than its nominal yield.

B. its nominal yield is higher than its YTM.

C. its nominal yield and its YTM are the same.

D. its YTM is higher than its current yield.

55. All of the following are features of ETFs EXCEPT

    A.   redeemed by the issuer.

    B.   typically lower fees than closed-end company shares.

    C.   initially capitalized through a public IPO.

    D.   often track an index or other benchmark.

56. Which of the following options positions obligates an investor to purchase stock?

    A.   Long put

    B.   Long call

    C.   Short put

    D.   Short call

57. An investor has 100 shares of XYZ stock at $90 per share. After a 3-for-1 split, the investor can expect to own

    A.   300 shares at $30 per share.

    B.   300 shares at $90 per share.

    C.   100 shares at $90 per share.

    D.   100 shares at $30 per share.

58. XYZ Inc. declares a $0.30 dividend payable on Monday, August 15, to all shareholders of record as of Monday, August 8. When is the ex-dividend date for a regular way trade in the stock?

    A.   Friday, August 5

    B.   Thursday, August 4

    C.   Wednesday, August 3

    D.   Tuesday, August 2

59. Which of the following is a key difference between a Traditional IRA and a Roth IRA?

    A.   Roth IRAs are not available to everyone with earned income, but Traditional IRAs are.

    B.   Annual contribution limits are higher in Traditional IRAs

    C.   A 10% penalty for withdrawals before age 59 ½ exists only in a Traditional IRA, not a Roth IRA

D.   The annual contribution deadline is different

60. In a 401(k) with a Roth account option, how are employer matching contributions allocated?

   A.   To the Roth account only

   B.   To the regular 401(k) only

   C.   To either the regular 401(k) or Roth account, at the employer's option

   D.   To either the regular 401(k) or Roth account, at the employee's option

61. The SEC has declared a new public offering effective. This indicates that

   E.   the SEC has verified the issuer's information.

   F.   the SEC approves of the new issue.

   G.   the SEC recommends the issuer's securities for purchase.

   H.   the SEC has cleared the issuance for public sale.

62. An unsecured bond is also known as a(n)

   I.   collateral trust bond.

   J.   indenture.

   K.   private activity bond.

   L.   debenture.

63. The Securities Investor Protection Corporation (SIPC) protects customers from

   M.   issuer bankruptcy.

   N.   market loss.

   O.   identity theft compromising customer accounts or the broker-dealer.

   P.   broker-dealer financial failure.

64. A customer must sign and return the options account agreement

   Q.   at or prior to placing the initial trade in the account.

   R.   at or prior to the approval of the account.

   S.   within 15 calendar days of account approval.

T. within 15 calendar days of placing the initial trade.

65. An 80 -year-old individual would be least likely to purchase a

    U. treasury bond.

    V. hedge fund.

    W. money market fund.

    X. bank CD.

66. Henry and Jennifer, a married couple, have a net worth of $800,000, excluding home equity. Their income has been about $250,000 for several years. Are they eligible to participate in a private placement of securities as accredited investors?

    A. No, because they meet neither test

    B. Yes, because they meet both tests

    C. Yes, because they meet the net worth test

    D. Yes, because they meet the income test

67. Which of the following statements is TRUE regarding the value of variable contract annuity units?

    Y. It is linked to the performance of the insurance company's general account

    Z. It is determined by a formula specified in the annuity contract

    AA. It fluctuates based on the performance of separate account assets

    BB. It is fixed at the time of the contract's annuitization

68. Passive losses generated by a limited partnership may be used to reduce which of the following?

    CC. Capital gains from the sale of appreciated investments only

    DD. Both ordinary income and passive income

    EE. Ordinary income only

    FF. Passive income only

69. Investors that purchase high quality fixed income investments for retirement income are most concerned with

GG. economic risk.

HH. inflation risk.

II. principal risk.

JJ. credit risk.

70. The "third market" is a marketplace where

KK. listed securities trade in the OTC market.

LL. listed securities trade in their primary listing venue.

MM.   OTC securities trade in a foreign market.

NN. OTC securities trade on a stock exchange.

71. The money supply will tighten based on which of these techniques of monetary policy?

OO. The Federal Reserve reduces the reserve requirement

PP. The Federal Reserve purchases government securities from primary dealers

QQ. The U.S. Government decreases government spending

RR. The Federal Reserve increases the discount rate

72. What type of order should Martin enter if his objective is to buy 500 shares of Cisco stock as soon as possible at the best price available?

SS. Limit

TT. Market

UU. Trailing stop

VV. Good-till-cancelled

73. An individual contacts her financial representative to sell her mutual fund shares. The price she will receive is

WW.   the next calculated POP price.

XX. the asked price at the close of the trading day.

YY. the next calculated NAV price.

ZZ. the market price at the time the order is entered.

74. The regulatory element of continuing education must be completed on the

AAA.   third anniversary of initial registration, and every second year thereafter.

BBB.   second anniversary of initial registration, and every third year thereafter.

CCC.   second anniversary of initial registration, and every two years thereafter.

DDD.   first anniversary of initial registration, and every two years thereafter.

75. When must the brokerage firm deliver a customer confirmation to the customer?

EEE.   When an order is placed

FFF.   Within three days of trade date

GGG.   Upon the customer's request

HHH.   At or before completion of each transaction

Mock Exam 3 - Questions

1. Each member broker-dealer is required to have a principal executive monitoring the firm's adherence to SRO as well as State and Federal laws and regulations, known as the firm's

   A. CCO

   B. COO

   C. CEO

   D. Business Continuity contact person

2. In the industry, the term 'Blue Chip' most often is associated with:

   A. stocks that outperform GDP

   B. stocks that outperform the CPI

   C. stocks that consistently produce income and modest growth over long periods of time

   D. All of the above

3. When a customer places a purchase order for an NYSE stock and the trade is reported at a price which is different than the actual transaction price,

   A. the client pays the price initially reported

   B. the client is given the better price

   C. the trade goes through at a price approved by FINRA

   D. the client pays the price at which the trade was executed

4. ETPs (exchange-traded products) generally include:

   A. ELNs

   B. ETFs

   C. ETNs

   D. any of the above fit this category

5. Under what conditions, if any, may an agent of a broker-dealer share in the profits and losses of a customer's account?

   A. only if the sharing is in direct proportion to the financial contribution made by the agent to the account

B. under no circumstances

C. only if it is a discretionary account

D. only with permission from an SRO such as FINRA

6. Under the Internal Revenue Code as it pertains to traditional individual retirement accounts (IRA),

A. required minimum distributions must begin upon reaching age 59 ½ years of age.

B. required minimum distributions must begin upon reaching age 70 ½ years of age.

C. required minimum distributions may begin upon reaching age 70 ½ years of age.

D. required minimum distributions may begin upon reaching age 59 ½ years of age.

7. The agency in charge of maintaining a list of individuals and institutions for which opening a brokerage account may be prohibited or restricted is known as:

A. CTR

B. Treasury

C. OFAC

D. SAR

8. In order for a registered representative to maintain their securities license on an ongoing basis, which of the following properly states the CE requirements?

A. passing a regulatory element CE exam within 2 years of their anniversary date.

B. passing a firm element CE exam every 3 years after their anniversary date.

C. passing a regulatory element CE exam within 3 years of their anniversary date.

D. passing a firm element CE exam within 1 year of their anniversary date.

9. When an agent engages in securities activities outside the scope of their broker-dealer,

A. the agent must update their Form U-4 within 30 days.

B. the agent must disclose this activity to their principal within 24 hours.

C. the agent must show they understand the suitability requirements of the securities being sold.

D. the agent is in violation of FINRA rules prohibiting selling away.

10. A large institutional client of yours has discussed their imminent intent to place a very large purchase order for the stock of XYZ. As the agent of record, you place an order immediately in your own account prior to placing the client's order.

A. this is known as front-running

B. this is a manipulative act

C. this is only permitted with permission of your principal

D. this is only permitted with written authorization from the client

11. That most basic tenet of a suitability determination is the:

A. follow the customer's instructions

B. only recommend that which is suitable for yourself

C. written supervisory procedures of your firm

D. know your customer rule

12. Making cold calls to prospects in accordance with the telemarketing consumer protection act may only be done:

A. between 8 am and 9 pm in your time zone

B. during trading hours in your time zone

C. between 8 am and 9 pm in the prospect's time zone

D. between 9 am and 8 pm in the prospect's time zone

13. A customer of a brokerage firm must receive a customer account statement with which of the following frequencies?

I.   Monthly

II.   Weekly if there has been any activity in the account

III. A minimum of at least quarterly

IV.   Monthly if there has been any activity in the account

A. I and II

B. II and III

C. I and IV

D. III and IV

14. United States government budgetary and taxation policies are best described as:

A. fiscal policy

B. keynesian policies

C. monetary policy

D. legislative policies

15. When one of the individuals in an account opened as Tenants in Common dies, their share of the account:

A. avoids probate

B. reverts to the surviving co-tenant

C. is subject to distribution in accordance with SEC Rule 15c3-3

D. goes to their estate

16. Regulation S-P principally deals with:

A. cybersecurity requirements

B. protection of privacy and identity information of clients

C. abuse of senior and elderly clients

D. disclosure of an introducing relationship to a clearing brokerage firm

17. All states have a securities Administrator whose job it is to enforce the securities laws of their state. All Administrators are part of an organization known as:

A. FINRA

B. the SEC

C. the SROs

D. NASAA

18. When a commercial bank elects to borrow short-term, often overnight, loans from another commercial bank, these loans are done at an interest rate known as the:

A. discount rate

B. prime rate

C. fed funds rate

D. call loan rate

19. The US economy has traditionally performed in a way described by economists and analysts as the business cycle. When an economy that has been operating a peak efficiency begins to slow down, which phase of the cycle is the economy entering?

A. contraction

B. recovery

C. expansion

D. trough

20. It is not unusual for a broker-dealer to fill a customer order for an NYSE stock as principal out of inventory in lieu of wiring it to the floor the exchange.

A. this is a second market transaction

B. this is a 4th market transaction

C. this is a 1st market transaction

D. this is a 3rd market transaction

21. Though there are numerous business sectors in the US economy, companies generally fall into three distinct categories:

A. large cap; mid-cap; small-cap

B. passive; active; tactical

C. cyclical; defensive; growth

D. conservative; moderate; speculative

22. In the business of underwriting, when a firm adopts a firm commitment, it is acting as a:

A. wholesaler

B. broker

C. distributor

D. dealer

23. Not all corporate securities offerings are required to be registered with the SEC. An offering done under Regulation D is often called:

A. a private placement

B. a limited partnership DPP

C. an emerging growth company offering

D. an intrastate exemption

24. When the US dollar weakens,

A. imports from foreign countries tend to increase

B. exports to foreign countries tend to increase

C. the FRB will engage in QE policy

D. US trade deficit will tend to rise

25. One of the primary risks associated with mortgage backed securities is prepayment risk. This tends to present itself when

A. inflation is increasing

B. the Fed reduces interest rates

C. the dollar is strong

D. none of the above

26. Among the most significant differences between an open-end investment management company and a unit investment trust is that:

A. the open-end company has a net asset value and a UIT does not.

B. the open-end company issues redeemable securities and the UIT does not.

C. the UIT has a fixed portfolio and the open-end company does not.

D. they require different FINRA licenses for an agent to sell them.

27. Single stock, or single sector, risk is more generally in the category described as:

A. systematic risk

B. market risk

C. non-systematic risk

D. economic risk

28. Diversification is a very effective way for an investor to mitigate:

A. business risk

B. market risk

C. monetary risk

D. longevity risk

29. Many folks living across the country choose to participate in their state's 529 college savings plan. These investment programs are generally referred to by FINRA as:

A. municipal fund securities

B. LGIPs

C. pre-paid tuition plans

D. UGMA or UTMA

30. As interest rates rise, which of the below will change the least in price?

A. T-bills

B. T-notes

C. T-bonds

D. their prices react roughly the same amount

31. Your client wishes to make a substantial investment in a mutual fund your firm is offering. In order to qualify for a reduced sales load, they sign a letter of intent which gives them:

A. a year to comply with the breakpoint level

B. 13 months to comply with the breakpoint level

C. 90 days to comply with the breakpoint level

D. an obligation to comply with the rules regarding breakpoint qualification

32. Choose from among the below ratings the one which is the higher credit rating in the speculative category

as defined by Standard & Poors rating service would be:

A. AAA

B. BB+

C. Ba1

D. CCC

33. The security instrument most often associated with enabling a US investor to facilitate trading in foreign stock is:

A. ADR

B. GDP

C. CMO

D. Forward contracts

34. The writer of an option contract is said to have:

A. a long option position

B. a long stock position

C. a short option position

D. a short stock position

35. Absent exceptional circumstances, NASDAQ trades during business hours are reported within:

A. 15 minutes of the trade

B. 1 minute of the trade

C. 30 seconds of the trade

D. 10 seconds of the trade

36. An NYSE listed corporation has outstanding preferred stock with a cumulative provision and a $5.00 annual dividend. If the earnings over the past two years have led to the Board of Directors declaring a $3.00 preferred dividend two years ago and a $2.00 dividend last year, in order that a common dividend may be paid for the current year:

A. Dividends in arrears of $5.00 must be paid to the preferred

B. Preferred stockholders must be paid $10 per share

C. Preferred stockholders need to be paid their current $ 5.00 dividend

D. None of the above is accurate.

37. When an investor writes a covered call, the client's profit and loss potential on that position becomes:

A. Unlimited loss and limited profit

B. Unlimited loss and unlimited profit

C. Limited loss and unlimited profit

D. Limited loss and limited profit

38. When the term 'shelf registration' is used, it typically refers to:

A. Registering securities with the SEC in anticipation of a future offering.

B. Registering securities with the SEC and selling part of the registered securities immediately and reserving the remaining securities for sale at a later time.

C. Filing a notice with the SEC of the Issuer's intent to file a registration statement in the next 90 days.

D. An offering which began but due to lackluster public interest, was put 'on the shelf' for a period not to exceed 30 days to see if investor interest picked up.

39. When institutional investment managers open brokerage accounts at several clearing broker-dealers, those clearing broker-dealers process the transactions and have the back-office clearing and processing handled through a single broker-dealer. This firm is identified in the SEC and FINRA regulations as a:

A. Floor Broker

B. Registered Trader

C. Prime broker

D. Omnibus firm

40. When a Board declares a cash dividend, the order of dates beginning with that announcement date is:

I.   Declaration date

II. Payment date

III. Record date

IV. Ex-dividend date

A. I, III, IV, II

B. II, III, IV, I

C. I, II, IV, III

D. I, IV, III, II

41. A market maker is quoting a stock at 23.15 – 23.30. If the firm fails to honor its quote for at least one round lot on both sides of the market,

A. It will be guilty of a manipulative and deceptive act.

B. It will be guilty of a backing away violation.

C. It will be involuntarily removed as a market maker in that stock for a period of one month.

D. This is not a violation.

42. When investors put their capital at risk, they rely upon the input and advice of their financial advisors, persons associated with a broker-dealer who have been trained in the field of investments and investment risks. As a concept, hedging has its primary purpose:

A. Increasing maximum potential profits while eliminating the risk of loss.

B. Mitigating maximum potential loss.

C. Limiting loss as well as limited profit.

D. Reducing potential taxes on an investment.

43. NASDAQ market makers wishing to increase the ADTV (average daily trading volume) they handle in those stocks:

A. May publish positive research reports about those issuers

B. May instruct their registered reps to recommend those issues to their customers in greater amounts.

C. May pay other brokerage firms to direct trades in those issues to the market maker for execution.

D. None of the above are permitted activities

44. A client of yours purchased 1000 shares of RAL common stock on Monday, February 11th in a cash account at a CMV of $115 per share. The next day the stock moves to $128 on a very favorable news report and the client places an order to sell the 1000 shares at the market. On the Reg. T payment date the client has not paid for the purchase and asks that liquidation proceeds be used to cover the cost of the purchase.

A. This is free-riding, a violation of Reg. T

B. This is a variation of front-running, a fraudulent act.

C. This is referred to as trading ahead.

D. Your firm will begin an investigation into the probability that this client had access to inside information prior to the announcement of the favorable news.

45. A short call is:

A. An option contract where the investor has a contractual obligation, for the duration of the contract, to deliver the underlying instrument at the strike price upon exercise.

B. An option contract where the investor has a contractual obligation until expiry to purchase the underlying instrument at the exercise price upon exercise.

C. An option contract where the investor has borrowed a call option from an investor with a long position and sold it short in anticipation of a decline in the option premium prior to expiry.

D. An option contract where the investors has the right to purchase the underlying instrument at any time prior to option expiration at the designated strike price.

46. Allowable ways to qualify for a breakpoint when purchasing front-end load mutual funds include:

I.   Exchange or conversion privilege with a fund family

II. Reinvesting dividends and/or capital gains distributions under an LOI.

III. 13-month LOI

IV. ROA – rights of accumulation

A. All of the above

B. II, III, and IV

C. III and IV

D. III only

47. Each of the below business enterprises exhibit flow-through of tax and related consequences except:

A. DPP

B. LLC

C. Sub S

D. C corp

48. Depreciation write-offs represent which of the following?

A. An estimate of the loss in value of a tangible asset over time.

B. An IRS mandated percentage allowable annual non-cash charge against revenues

C. A subtraction from the computation of corporate cash flow.

D. A tax deduction for the loss in value due to extraction or removal.

49. Every FINRA member firm must have in place a Business Continuity Plan which addresses:

A. How the firm will continue operations if and when the firm is sold

B. How the firm will continue operations if and when the firm becomes subject to a SIPC proceedings.

C. How customers of the firm will be able to access their accounts and assets during a disaster or pandemic which has made normal operations infeasible

D. How the firm's hiring practices will comport with Department of Labor rulings in a proper and timely way.

50. A candidate who fails the SIE exam three times and has waited the six-month moratorium period is preparing to take the exam for the fourth time. Which of the following is true?

A. The candidate will be required to pass the exam or wait for a 30-day wait period before a 5th attempt.

B. The candidate will be told by FINRA that a one-year moratorium period will be put in place.

C. The candidate will be given a more difficult version of the exam.

D. The candidate will have to wait another six-months if the exam is failed on the 4th try.

51. If a mutual fund purchaser signs a letter of intent in order to take advantage of a breakpoint discount, how long does he have to buy enough shares to reach the breakpoint?

A. 25 months

B. 13 months

C. 9 months

D. 90 days

52. Front-running refers to the practice of:

A. Inter-positioning

B. Trading ahead of research reports

C. Trading ahead of a customer's block order

D. Trading ahead of marketable customer orders

53. Which of the following investors would be most subject to inflationary risk?

   A. Kim, whose portfolio is a mix of blue chip and small cap securities

   B. Bill, whose portfolio is composed primarily of U.S. Treasury bonds

   C. Sarah, 75% of whose portfolio is made up of dividend-paying stocks

   D. Steve, whose portfolio consists mainly of U.S. Treasury bills and bank CDs

54. Of the following, which is the correct definition for open market operations?

   A. When the Fed buys and sells foreign bonds on the secondary market

   B. When the Fed buys and sells foreign bonds on the primary market

   C. When the Fed buys and sells U.S. treasury bonds on the primary market

   D. When the Fed buys and sells U.S. treasury bonds on the secondary market

55. Limited liability means that a common shareholder:

   A. Cannot be charged any more than a designated amount in addition to his initial investment

   B. Can never lose an amount in addition to his entire investment

   C. Is guaranteed to lose no less than a designated percentage of his investment

   D. Can never lose his entire investment

56. Blake goes long 1 ABC Jan 40 put @ 7 when the market is 42. 7 months later, Blake closes the contract at intrinsic value when the market is at 39. What is the gain or loss?

   A. -$600

   B. $600

   C. $700

   D. $500

57. Which of the following bonds will rise the furthest in price when interest rates fall?

A. 30 year 10% mortgage bond

B. 10 year 4% Treasury bond

C. 14 year 6% debenture

D. 8 year 5% revenue bond

58. A Clearing Firm is

A. The company that handles orders to buy and sell securities and maintains custody of securities and other assets.

B. The company that acts as an agent or principal in a securities transaction and charges commissions or markups.

C. The company that quotes both a buy and a sell price in a security held in inventory, hoping to make a profit on the bid-offer spread.

D. The company that changes the name on a stock certificate for transactions and records it on the official master shareholder listing.

59. Which entity conducts the USA's monetary policy to promote maximum employment, stable prices, and moderate long-term interest rates in the United States economy?

A. FDIC

B. SIPC

C. Department Of The Treasury

D. Federal Reserve

60. A checking account that is held at a regional bank is guaranteed by

A. Federal Reserve

B. MSRB

C. FDIC

D. FINRA

61. If inflation has been increasing at an increasing rate, which of the following actions might the Federal Reserve

Board take?

A. Decreasing interest rates

B. Increasing interest rates

C. Increasing the money supply

D. Lowering bank reserve requirements

62. Which of the following transactions takes place in the secondary market?

A. A customer places a trade to sell a stock and it is executed on the NASDAQ.

B. An institution transacts a 1 million share block in dark pool.

C. A broker dealer sells an OTCQX stock to a hedge fund.

D. A customer buys an IPO before it is listed on the NYSE.

63. The document released by the issuer of municipal securities for a primary offering that discloses material information is called the

A. Red Herring

B. Prospectus

C. Official Statement

D. Preliminary Prospectus

64. In the event of a corporate liquidation, which of the following has the highest priority to corporate assets?

A. Callable Preferred Stock

B. Convertible Bonds

C. Unsecured Debt

D. Secured Debt

65. A 3.5 % GO Municipal Bond last traded at 99. This bond is selling at

A. A premium

B. Its NAV

C. A discount

D. Par value

66. Which of the following is true of a new issue?

A. A broker-dealer can accept payment from a new customer only if the preliminary prospectus is amended.

B. A broker-dealer can accept payment from a new customer when the red herring is delivered.

C. A broker-dealer can accept payment from a new customer when the registration is effective.

D. A broker-dealer can accept payment from a new customer during and toward the end of the cooling off period.

67. A hedge fund manager that is long large cap US stocks in the fund's portfolio may hedge his risk by

A. Buying Russell 2000 index puts

B. Selling Russell 2000 index calls

C. Selling S&P 500 index calls

D. Buying S&P 500 index puts

68. Authorized stock is all of the following, except:

A. It is arbitrarily determined at the time of incorporation and may not be changed.

B. It is the maximum number of shares a company may sell.

C. It may be sold to investors to raise operating capital for the company.

D. It may be sold in total or in part when the company goes public.

69. ABC common stock declined dramatically in value over the last quarter but the dividend it declared for payment this quarter has remained the same. The dividend yield on the stock has:

A. Gone up as the price of ABC has fallen.

B. Not changed because the board has to declare the dividend amount.

C. Been fixed at the time of issuance.

D. Gone down because the yield is a stated rate.

70. A corporation may pay a dividend in which of the following ways? Choose the most complete response.

A. Stock of another company.

B. Cash.

C. Stock.

D. All of the above.

71. When is the interest on an EE savings bond paid?

A. Monthly.

B. Quarterly.

C. Annually.

D. When redeemed.

72. A syndicate has published a tombstone ad prior to the issue becoming effective. Which of the following must appear in the tombstone?

I.   A statement that the ad is not an offer to sell the securities.

II. No commitment statement.

III. Contact information.

IV. A statement that the registration has not yet become effective.

A. I and II.

B. II and III.

C. III and IV.

D. All of the above

73. Which of the following is NOT a type of offering?

A. Subsequent primary offering.

B. Combined offering.

C. Secondary offering.

D. Rule 149 offering.

74. Which of the following are true about an option?

I.   The two parties are known as the buyer and the seller. The money paid by the buyer of the option is known as the option's premium.

II. The buyer has bought the right to buy or sell the security depending on the type of option.

III. It is a contract between two parties that determines the time and place at which a security may be bought or sold.

IV. The seller has an obligation to perform under the contract, possibly to buy or sell the stock depending on the option involved.

  A. I, II, and IV.

  B. I, II, and III.

  C. II, III, and IV.

  D. I, II, III, and IV.

75. In which type of account does the nominal owner of the account enter all orders for the beneficial owner of the account?

  A. Discretionary account.

  B. Authorized account.

  C. Custodial account.

  D. Fiduciary account.

Mock Exam 4 - Questions

1. It may be necessary for a company to repurchase some of its stock, to increase its treasury stock, for which one of the following reasons:

   A. To increase the funding in the company's treasury.

   B. To allow the company to pay out smaller dividends.

   C. To reassure its investors that all is well.

   D. To maintain control of the company.

2. An investor owns 100 shares of XYZ 8% participating preferred stock. XYZ's common stock pays a quarterly dividend of $.25. How much will the investor earn each year in dividends?

   A. $900.

   B. $825.

   C. $180.

   D. $90.

3. An investor has purchased shares of a foreign company through an ADR. Which of the following is not true?

   A. The dividend will be paid in U.S. dollars.

   B. The investor is subject to currency risk.

   C. The ADR may represent one or more shares of the company's common stock.

   D. The investor may elect to exchange the ADR for the underlying common shares.

4. An investor would expect to realize the largest capital gain by buying bonds that are:

   A. Long-term when rates are high.

   B. Short-term when rates are low.

   C. Short-term when rates are high.

   D. Long-term when rates are low.

5. The type of bond that is secured by real estate is called a:

   A. Mortgage bond.

B. Real estate trust certificate.

C. Collateral trust certificate.

D. Equipment trust certificate.

6. XYZ has 8% subordinated debentures trading in the market place at $120. They are convertible into XYZ common stock at $25 per share. What is the parity price of the common stock?

   A. 31.

   B. 30.

   C. 29.

   D. 28.

7. When contrasting a corporate bond to a municipal bond of the same quality and maturity, you would observe which of the following?

   A. The corporate bond has a higher coupon rate.

   B. The municipal bond is more volatile.

   C. The corporate bond has a lower coupon rate.

   D. The corporate bond is more volatile.

8. An investor purchased a Treasury bond at 95.03. How much did he pay for the bond?

   A. $ 9,500.9375.

   B. $ 9,530.00.

   C. $ 953.00.

   D. $ 950.9375.

9. Which of the following could trade in the money market?

   A. A Treasury note issued nine years ago.

   B. Short-term equity.

   C. Newly issued options contracts.

   D. Newly issued corporate bonds.

10. Which of the following is NOT true of money market instruments?

A. They are issued by corporations with high credit ratings, and are thus considered safe.

B. They are highly liquid fixed-income securities.

C. They are a method used to obtain short-term financing.

D. They are considered risky because of short-term maturities.

11. Which one of the following interest rates is controlled by the Federal Reserve Board?

A. Federal funds rate.

B. Prime rate.

C. Discount rate.

D. Broker call loan rate.

12. The Federal Reserve Board sets all of the following except:

A. Governmental spending.

B. Reserve requirement.

C. Discount rate.

D. Monetary policy.

13. During a new issue registration, false information is included in the prospectus to buyers. Which of the following may be held liable to investors?

I.   People who signed the registration statement.

II.   Officers of the issuer.

III.   Syndicate members.

IV.   Accountants.

A. I and III.

B. I, II, and III.

C. I, III, and IV.

D. I, II, III, and IV.

14. A company doing a preemptive rights offering would most likely use what type of underwriting agreement?

A. Firm commitment.

B. Best efforts.

C. Standby.

D. All or none.

15. A corporation in your state wants to sell 1,000,000 shares of stock at $5 per share to investors. Which of the following is NOT true under Rule 147?

A. 80% of proceeds must be used in the state.

B. 80% of corporate assets must be located in the state.

C. 80% of the purchasers must be in the state.

D. 80% of the income must be derived from activity within the state.

16. A firm participating in the offering of a private placement may sell the private placement to no more than _____ nonaccredited investors in any 12-month period?

A. 15.

B. 35.

C. 6.

D. 12.

17. The city of Miami is seeking to raise $10 million through the sale of general obligation bonds to repair the high school's football field. The bonds are going to be issued ex-legal. Which of the following is correct?

A. The bonds' legal claim to the tax revenue is in doubt.

B. The bonds received no legal opinion.

C. The bonds received a qualified legal opinion.

D. The bonds received an unqualified legal opinion.

18. Which of the following is NOT a type of order?

I. Best efforts.

II. Mini/maxi.

III. Fill or kill.

IV. All or none.

    A. I and II.

    B. III and IV.

    C. II and IV.

    D. I and IV.

19. ABC Technologies, a very volatile stock, closes at $180 per share. Your customer has placed an order to sell 500 ABC at 165 stop limit 160 GTC. After the close, the company announces bad earnings and the stock opens at 145. What happened to your customer's order?

    A. It has been elected and has become a limit order.

    B. It has been canceled because the stock price is below the limit price.

    C. It has been canceled because the stock price is below the stop price.

    D. It has been elected and executed.

20. Your brokerage firm acts as a market maker for several high-volume stocks that are quoted on the Nasdaq. What is the firm's consideration for being a market maker?

    A. 5%.

    B. Spread.

    C. Fees.

    D. Commission.

21. The OCC is:

    A. Options Counseling Committee.

    B. Options Clearing Committee.

    C. Options and Claims Corporation.

    D. Options Clearing Corporation.

22. Your customer is long 100 shares of MSFT. The investor wants to protect the position without spending any additional money, what should he do?

    A. Buy a put.

118

B. Buy a call.

C. Sell a call.

D. Sell a put.

23. An investor wires $10,000 into his mutual fund on Tuesday, March 11, and the money is credited to his account at 3 p.m. He will be the owner of record on:

A. Tuesday, March 11.

B. Wednesday, March 12.

C. Tuesday, March 18.

D. Friday, March 14.

24. A mutual fund that assesses a charge to cover promotional expenses would be charging:

A. A balanced load.

B. A redemption charge.

C. A 12b-1 fee.

D. A contingent deferred sales charge.

25. A fixed annuity guarantees all of the following except:

A. Rate of return.

B. Income for life.

C. Protection from investment risk.

D. Protection from inflation.

26. An investor has placed a sum equal to 50% of the annual contribution limit into his traditional IRA. The investor is seeking to maximize his contributions to his retirement savings. Which of the following is correct?

A. The investor may only contribute to a traditional IRA if one has been established.

B. The investor may contribute a sum equal to 50% of the annual limit to a Roth IRA.

C. The investor may contribute 100% of the annual limit to a Roth IRA.

D. The investor may not contribute to a Roth IRA.

27. The maximum amount that a couple may contribute to their IRAs at any one time is:

A. 400% of the annual contribution limit.

B. 300% of the annual contribution limit.

C. 200% of the annual contribution limit.

D. 100% of the annual contribution limit.

28. A client who is 65 years old has invested $10,000 in a Roth IRA. It has now grown to $14,000. He plans to retire and take a lump sum distribution. He will pay taxes on:

A. $14,000.

B. $10,000.

C. $4,000.

D. $0.

29. Which of the following is NOT allowed as a joint account?

A. A registered representative and a spouse.

B. A registered representative and a customer.

C. A registered representative and his 16-year-old child.

D. A registered representative and a friend.

30. Which of the following is not a violation of the rules of conduct?

A. Recommending a mutual fund based on a pending dividend to an investor seeking income.

B. Showing a client the past performance of a mutual fund for the last 3 years since its inception.

C. Implying that FINRA has approved the firm.

D. Recommending a security because of its future price appreciation.

31. An investor has a conservative attitude towards investing and is seeking to invest $50,000 into an interest-bearing instrument that will provide current income and safety. You would most likely recommend which of the following?

A. Ginnie Mae pass-through certificate.

B. Bankers' acceptance.

C. Treasury bill.

D. Treasury STRIP.

32. You are the owner of a restaurant and you would like to have a guitarist play in the lounge on Saturday evenings. You have known your representative for 15 years and know her to be a great jazz guitarist. You think she would like to play and ask her if she is available to do so. She would have to notify which of the following before accepting your offer?

A. NYSE.

B. Her firm.

C. FINRA.

D. No one, because it is not securities related and she is on her own time.

33. An individual applying for registration with a FINRA member firm would be required to include which of the following on Form U4?

A. Educational background.

B. 5-year residence history.

C. A divorce.

D. 5-year employment history.

34. A firm has been taken to arbitration by a customer. The disputed amount is $47,400. Which of the following is true?

A. There will be a hearing, and the arbitrator's decision is final.

B. There will be a hearing, and the decision may be appealed.

C. There will be a hearing with up to three arbitrators.

D. There will not be a hearing, and the decision may not be appealed.

35. A testimonial by a compensated expert, citing the results she realized following a member's recommendations, must include which of the following?

I.   The name of the principal who approved the ad.

II. A statement detailing the expert's credentials.

III. A statement that the individual is a compensated spokesperson.

IV. A statement that past performance is not a guarantee of future performance.

A. I and II.

B. II, III, and IV.

C. I, II, and III.

D. All of the above.

36. You are the owner of a restaurant and you would like to have a guitarist play in the lounge on Saturday evenings. You have known your representative for 15 years and know her to be a great jazz guitarist. You think she would like to play and ask her if she is available to do so. She would have to notify which of the following before accepting your offer?

A. No one, because it is not securities related and she is on her own time.

B. Her firm.

C. NYSE.

D. FINRA.

37. Which act gave the NASD (now part of FINRA) the authority to regulate the OTC market?

A. The Securities Act of 1933.

B. The NASD Act of 1929.

C. The Maloney Act of 1938.

D. The Securities Act of 1934.

38. An investor is looking for a risk-free investment. An agent should recommend which of the following to this investor?

A. Bankers' acceptances.

B. Preferred stock.

C. Convertible preferred stock.

D. 90-day T-bill.

39. An investor has a conservative attitude toward investing and is seeking to invest $100,000 into an instrument that will provide current income and the most protection from interest rate risk. You would most likely

recommend which of the following?

A. A portfolio of T-bills.

B. Bankers' acceptance.

C. Treasury STRIP.

D. Ginnie Mae pass-through certificate.

40. A customer has a large position in GJH, a thinly traded stock whose share price has remained flat for some time. The customer contacts the agent and wants to sell his entire position. The customer is most subject to which of the following?

A. Credit risk.

B. Liquidity risk.

C. Execution risk.

D. Conversion risk.

41. Which of the following is true?

A. Broker dealers may not give gifts to the employees of other broker dealers.

B. A representative may not obtain outside employment because of the potential conflict of interest.

C. A client may not have a numbered account for his investment account.

D. Representatives and broker dealers may not disclose any information regarding a client to a third party without the client's expressed consent or a court order.

42. Which of the following accounts would not subject the account owner to required minimum distributions?

I.   A traditional IRA.

II.   A Roth IRA.

III. A joint account with survivorship rights.

IV.   A variable annuity.

A. I only.

B. I and III.

C. I, II, and III.

D. II, III and IV.

43. An investor who wishes to include a prior purchase of a mutual fund in a new letter of intent, wants to backdate the letter. Which of the following is correct?

A. He may do this within 3 months.

B. He may do this within 7 business days.

C. He may do this within 2 months.

D. He may do this within 1 month.

44. An investor with $20,000 invested in the XYZ growth fund is:

A. An owner of XYZ.

B. A stockholder in XYZ.

C. Both an owner of XYZ and an owner of an undivided interest in the XYZ growth portfolio.

D. An owner of an undivided interest in the XYZ growth portfolio.

45. You are long 10,000 shares of XYZ at 42 and are concerned about a market decline; you would like to take in some additional income. You should:

A. Sell 10 XYZ Oct 45 calls.

B. Sell 100 XYZ Oct 45 puts.

C. Sell 100 XYZ Oct 45 calls.

D. Sell 10 XYZ Oct 45 puts.

46. Which of the following issues standardized options?

A. Nasdaq.

B. Company.

C. OCC.

D. Exchanges.

47. Which of the following may NOT trade on the floor of the NYSE?

A. Allied member.

B. Two-dollar broker.

C. Commission house broker.

D. Regular member.

48. The state of Massachusetts is seeking to raise $300 million through the sale of revenue bonds to repair the roadways. Which of the following is correct?

A. The underwriters will be required to submit sealed bids.

B. The offering will be advertised in the daily bond buyer.

C. These bonds will be issued through a negotiation.

D. These bonds will be subject to a statutory debt limit.

49. For an insider to sell unregistered stock under an exemption from registration with the SEC, Form 144, Notice of Offering, which contains certain information, must be filed with the SEC. The insider can sell securities during the period of time in which the notice of offering is effective, which is:

A. 12 months.

B. 90 days.

C. 60 days.

D. 6 months.

50. A red herring given to a client during the cooling-off period will contain all of the following, except:

A. Use of proceeds.

B. Proceeds to the company.

C. A notice that all the information is subject to change.

D. Biographies of officers and directors.

51. An investor buys 100 shares of XYZ 7% convertible preferred stock which are convertible into XYZ common stock at $20 per share. How many shares of common stock are there upon conversion?

A. 5,000.

B. 500.

C. 400.

D. 5.

52. Which of the following is not true regarding American Depositary Receipts (ADRs)?

A. Each ADR represents 100 shares of foreign stock, and the ADR holder may request delivery of the foreign shares.

B. They are receipts of ownership of foreign shares being held abroad in a U.S. bank.

C. The foreign country may issue restrictions on the foreign ownership of stock.

D. ADR holders have the right to vote and to receive dividends that the foreign corporation declares for shareholders.

53. An investor holding an 8% subordinated debenture will receive how much at maturity?

A. Depends on the purchase price.

B. $1,080.

C. $1,040.

D. $1,000.

54. A company you own common stock in has just filed for bankruptcy. As a shareholder, you will have the right to receive:

A. New common shares in the reorganized company.

B. A percentage of your original investment.

C. The par value of the common shares.

D. Your proportional percentage of residual assets.

55. An ABC corporate bond is quoted at 110 and is convertible into ABC common at 20 per share parity. Price for the stock is:

A. 24.

B. 23.

C. 22.

D. 21.

56. Which of the following municipal issues would most likely have more than one source of revenue?

A. Bonds issued by the county to improve the municipal courthouse.

B. Bonds issued by the state to cover general working expenses.

C. Bonds issued by a turnpike authority to improve roads.

D. Bonds issued by a town to improve school buildings.

57. Your customer buys a U.S. T-bond at 103.16. How much did he pay for the bond?

A. $10,316.00.

B. 1,035.00.

C. $103.16.

D. $1,031.60.

58. The money market is a place where issuers go to:

A. Obtain short-term financing.

B. Obtain long-term financing.

C. Exchange money market instruments to their mutual benefit.

D. Offer higher interest rates for a higher yield.

59. The government has two tools it can use to try to influence the direction of the economy. They are:

A. Prime rate policy and fiscal policy.

B. Fiscal policy and money market policy.

C. Monetary policy and prime rate policy.

D. Monetary policy and fiscal policy.

60. XYZ has just gone public and is quoted on the Nasdaq Capital Market securities market. Any investor who buys XYZ must get a prospectus for how long?

A. 60 days.

B. 45 days.

C. 30 days.

D. 25 days.

61. Rule 145 covers which of the following?

A. Changes in par value.

B. Reverse splits.

C. Stock swaps.

D. Stock splits.

62. The city of Chicago is seeking to raise $100 million through the sale of general obligation bonds and is seeking an underwriter for the issue. Which of the following is correct?

A. The city is looking to the lower true interest cost to finance the issue.

B. The issue will be underwritten on a best efforts basis if the city's bonds are not in high demand.

C. The issue must be advertised and provide terms for bidding.

D. The issue will be awarded through a negotiation.

63. Which of the following subjects the investor to unlimited risk?

A. Converting a bond into the underlying common stock.

B. Selling stock short.

C. Selling common stock long.

D. Buying a speculative bond.

64. Which of the following are bearish?

I.   Put seller.

II.   Call seller.

III. Put buyer.

IV.   Call buyer.

A. I and II.

B. II and III.

C. II and IV.

D. III and IV.

65. A mutual fund has been seeking to attract new customers to invest in its growth fund. They have been running an advertising campaign that markets them as a diversified mutual fund. How much of any one company may they own?

A. 10%.

B. 9%.

C. 5%.

D. 15%.

66. A no-load mutual fund may charge a 12B-1 fee that is:

A. Less than .25 of 1% of the POP.

B. Less than .25 of 1% of the NAV.

C. Up to .25 of 1% of the NAV.

D. Up to .25 of 1% of the POP.

67. An investor has deposited $100,000 into a qualified retirement account over a 10-year period. The value of the account has grown to $175,000 and the investor plans to retire and take a lump sum withdrawal. The investor will pay:

A. Ordinary income taxes on the $100,000 and capital gains on the $75,000.

B. Ordinary income taxes on the whole $175,000.

C. Ordinary income taxes on the $75,000 only.

D. Capital gains tax on $75,000 only.

68. A customer calls in asking about how to put money aside for his children. He wants to open a custodial account for his two children, Bobby and Sue. What should you recommend?

A. Open two accounts for the two children, with him being the custodian on one and his wife being custodian on the other, as one parent may only be custodian for one child.

B. Open two accounts for both children, with him and his wife as custodian.

C. Open two accounts, one for each child, with he or his wife as custodians for both or for either.

D. Open one account immediately for both children.

69. An investor gets advance notice of a research report being issued and enters an order to purchase the security that is the subject of the research report. This is known as:

A. Trading ahead.

B. Advance trading.

C. Insider trading.

D. Front running.

70. Which of the following is true?

 A. A registered representative may not use the pending dividend payment as the sole basis for recommending a stock purchase.

 B. If an investor buys shares just prior to the ex date, he will have his investment money returned.

 C. After an investor's money is returned, the investor is still liable for taxes on the dividend amount.

 D. All of the above.

71. As it relates to a member firm conducting business with the public, all of the following are violations, except:

 A. Failing to execute a customer's order for a speculative security.

 B. Charging a customer a larger than normal commission for executing a specific order.

 C. Printing "FINRA" in large type on business cards.

 D. Stating that a new issue has been approved for sale by the SEC.

72. At a member firm, which of the following must be registered?

 A. A back-office margin clerk who assists the head of the margin department.

 B. A corporate officer whose sole function is to act as liaison between the board of directors and management.

 C. A receptionist who takes messages from customers inquiring about their accounts.

 D. A part-time sales assistant who occasionally takes verbal orders from customers.

73. According to Rule 135, as it relates to generic advertising, which of the following is NOT true?

 A. The ad may contain information about the performance of past recommendations.

 B. The ad may describe the nature of the investment company's business.

 C. The ad may contain information about the services a company offers.

 D. The ad may contain information about exchange privileges.

74. A FINRA member has failed to receive a stock certificate in good form from the selling FINRA firm. Which FINRA bylaw defines good delivery?

 A. Code of Procedure.

 B. Rules of Fair Practice.

C. Uniform Practice Code.

D. Code of Arbitration.

75. An investor who may lose part or all of his investment is subject to which of the following?

A. Market risk.

B. Credit risk.

C. Capital risk.

D. Reinvestment risk.

Mock Exam 1 - Answers and Rationales

1. A: The Act of '34 created the SEC.

2. B: The SEC reviews the information in a registration statement, it does not approve or disapprove of the information, nor does it guarantee the accuracy of the information disclosures. Therefore no sales agent can say to a prospect that these are 'government approved' securities.

3. D: SIPC was set up to protect customer ACCOUNTS in the event of a broker-dealer bankruptcy, not protect investments against loss. Be careful of the wording in this question. Cash & securities in customer accounts are 'insured' up to $500,000 in the event the B/D goes bankrupt and the cash and securities can't be located and properly returned to the customer.

4. C: Federal securities laws typically supersede State laws.

5. A: Since the 'money market' includes short term debt instruments only, and since ADRs represent ownership (equity) in foreign stocks, ADRs are not debt.

6. C: Going public means sharing equity ownership (common stock) with public investors, for the first time (Initial public offering, IPO).

7. D: Whether one considers answers A, B, or C partially accurate, the last answer, D is the most complete therefore best answer.

8. B: This is one of the functions of a Transfer Agent. Registrars make sure that a company does not issue more shares than authorized in the Charter.

9. C: You cannot lose more than you've put at risk. A common stockholder cannot be held liable for any debts of the corporation, therefore they have limited liability.

10. C: Splitting a stock provides each shareholder with more shares and the CMV (current market value) of the stock will decline proportionately. Because of the reduced price in the market, it becomes more 'affordable.'

11. B: Stock dividends are not Cash dividends – they are dividends in the form of additional shares.

12. D: All three are correct – in fact, Regular and Statutory are the same.

13. D: Call option contracts go 'in the money' (intrinsic value) when the current market value of the underlying security exceeds the exercise price (strike price) of the option. If a call option's exercise price is $20, and the underlying stock is trading at $25, the intrinsic value of the call option is $5.

14. B: Since with a Zero coupon instrument there is no annual income to 'reinvest,' Zeroes have no reinvestment risk.

15. B: Exchange traded funds trade on exchanges at market prices determined by supply and demand – the same as regular corporate stocks.

16. C: Variable annuities sell 'accumulation units' to purchasers, whose price each day is based upon the 4 pm net asset value of the separate account.

17. B: The maximum maturity is 9 months or 270 days.

18. C: This SIE exam enables the candidate to take one of several different FINRA registered reps exam.

19. C: Regulation T does not permit margin under normal circumstances on Option contracts.

20. B: Buying broad-based Index Put options will provide a hedge against the decline in the broad market.

21. B: The best (inside) bid is the price at which a client's liquidation (sell) order will be executed.

22. A: Market making firms post firm quotes during the trading day at which they are obligating themselves to do business with other firms as well as retail customers.

23. C: The more actively traded a stock (high volume), the narrower the spread between the bid and ask prices.

24. C: The FINRA markup markdown and commission policy does not apply to new issues as well as municipal bonds --- MSRB has its own such policy.

25. A: Syndicate implies a firm commitment; group implies best efforts.

26. B: Stabilizing implies keeping the price steady, which SEC allows in a new issue if done in accordance with strict guidelines of SEC---anti-manipulation guidelines.

27. C: SHO are the first 3 letters of the word 'short.' Answer C. best describes the basics of this regulation.

28. B: SIPC was never intended to guarantee customers against investment loss. It's an insurance program providing ½ million dollars of account insurance in the event a customer's brokerage firm goes bankrupt, with the maximum CASH coverage the same as bank FDIC coverage: $250K.

29. D: Investors seeking 'tax shelter' or 'tax advantage' are often suitable for the flow through benefits of DPPs (direct participation program--- limited partnerships).

30. A: Defensive: stable, utilities, basic food, the basic needs of life, these are NOT growth industries.

31. B: When an investor shorts/writes/sells a put option, they agree to be OBLIGATED to BUY the underlying instrument at the strike price.

32. C: NYSE hours and CBOE hours are the same. 9:30 to 4 ET for the NYSE is the same as 8:30 to 3:00 CT. Make sure you KNOW your time zones!

33. A: The term 'STOCK' dividend tells you this is a distribution, NOT of cash, but of more shares of STOCK.

34. B: A written allegation: this is formally known as a complaint.

35. A: Pink sheets: the Pinks: the Pink quotes: All these terms in your textbook speak of thinly traded, closely-held, low daily volume stocks, where liquidity is not especially present when compared to NYSE and NASDAQ stocks.

36. D: The stock split lowers the market price of a stock, which makes buying a round lot (100 sh.) more 'affordable.'

37. D: Each of these when associated with a bond issue makes the bond more attractive from a client's point of view.

38. B: SEC was formed in 1934.

39. D: Only the closed-end investment company trades at supply & demand pricing on an Exchange, and has no specific relationship to the fund's underlying asset value.

40. B: The 'trick' with this question is that anytime a company is selling NEW previously unissued shares from their Authorized shares maximum, those shares are NEW ---- Primary distribution means the shares being sold are NEW, never before issued, not previously owned by anyone.

41. A: The terms 'clearing' and 'carrying' have to do with a brokerage firm's performance of certain functions most other firms are not permitted to do, such as have physical possession and custody of customers' cash and securities.

42. D: Pre-emptive Rights entitle a corporate shareholder to purchase shares in an additional share offering at a favorable below market price. Warrants enable the holder of the warrant to buy more shares at an exercise price which when first set, tends to be higher than CMV at that time. Warrants are normally quite long term whereas rights typically expire in 30 days or less. Both are tradable on organized stock exchanges, such as the NYSE.

43. D: Each of these answers is a true statement.

44. B: Though a very simplistic way of describing Keynesian theory, it focuses on government taxation and spending policies, which are fiscal in nature. Answer A would be more appropriate if we were asking about monetary policies, which would be the work of the Federal Reserve.

45. B: The term Secondary Offering is used to describe a situation in which already-issued shares are being resold into the marketplace, usually by insiders, officers, and directors of a company. The shares being sold are NOT new shares coming from the company. A follow-on offering, also called an APO (additional public offering) is where a company is issuing and selling more new shares to the public.

46. C: M&A means mergers and acquisitions. This department assists companies in their efforts to

buy another company or sell their company to an interested buyer.

47. C: A client who owns stock is exposed to 100% loss of invested principal, unless the client engages is one of a number of strategies designed to mitigate/reduce the risk of loss. One such strategy is the sell stop order, in which the client picks a price at which he or she will exit/liquidate their stock position if the stock falls to that price level, 'stopping' the loss from getting any worse.

48. A: Any investor who writes a call or a put option, also known as selling an option, also known as 'shorting' an option, is obligated to perform in accordance with the terms of the contract, but only if the option is exercised by the person who had purchased the option, referred to as the holder of the option, or the long option position.

49. B: A notice of sale is an advertisement published by a municipality in order to get bids from interested broker-dealers who wish to underwrite the sale of that issuer's upcoming bond offering. The other answers are different names for documents which make full disclosure to purchases of securities.

50. C: Securities Investor Protection Act of 1970 created an insurance entity called the Securities Investor Protection Corporation. Its purpose is to provide protection to customers of bankrupt brokerage firms in the event the customers' cash and or securities have not been found during the bankruptcy proceedings. It is not investment insurance. Once you are finished, click the button below. Any items you have not completed will be marked incorrect.

51. D: The regulatory element of continuing education requires that all registered persons complete a computer-based training session within 120 days of the person's second registration anniversary and every three years thereafter. The content of the regulatory element is determined and provided by FINRA and is appropriate to the class of registered representative or principal. If a person does not complete the regulatory element during the prescribed period, the person's license will become inactive, and they will not be able to perform any of the activities that require registration, and they will not be compensated for any of those activities.

52. B: The strike price for a call option is the price at which the call seller is obligated to sell the underlying security to the call holder if the option is exercised. When the call option hits the strike price, it is said to be in the money; however, the call holder is not obligated to buy the underlying securities when they reach the strike price. Additionally, the strike price added to the option's premium, and not simply the strike price, is the breakeven point for both the holder and writer of a call option. Finally, the strike price for a put option, and not a call option, is the price at which the call writer must buy the underlying securities from the call holder when the put is exercised.

53. A: Contributions to a traditional IRA are usually made with pre-tax dollars, and thus they are taxed upon withdrawal. Additionally, although earnings in an IRA grow tax free, they are taxed upon withdrawal. Taxation of both pre-tax contributions and earnings occurs at the investor's ordinary tax rate, and the investor's age has no bearing on whether or not his withdrawals will be taxed.

54. A: Instead of forming a syndicate, an underwriter may choose to form a selling group. A selling group member has no obligation to buy the bonds. The financial risk of unsold bonds is borne entirely

by the managing underwriter when a selling group is used in lieu of a syndicate.

55. C: Treasury bonds pay interest semiannually (twice a year). In contrast, Treasury bills are bought at a discount and redeemed for par value at maturity. STRIPS are long-term zero coupon bonds consisting of U.S. Treasury securities. As zero-coupon bonds, they are bought at a discount and then redeemed for par value at maturity. Finally, treasury stock is issued stock that is repurchased by the issuing company. It is not issued by the U.S. Treasury and pays neither dividends nor interest.

56. D: HR-10 plans, also known as Keogh (pronounced key-o) plans, are retirement accounts created for smaller professional practices (like a dentist's office or law firm). Contributions to these plans are tax deductible, while distributions are fully taxable.

57. C: Common stock tends to outpace inflation (prices of goods and services rising), therefore investments in common stock can be used as a hedge (protection) against inflation. Fixed income investments (like preferred stock and bonds) are very susceptible to inflation and lose value when inflation rates rise.

58. C: Commercial paper will not exceed 270 days to maturity in order to avoid registration with the SEC. Registration is a costly endeavor, requiring legal counseling and significant amounts of paperwork. A corporation will avoid registration if possible.

59. B: A syndicate member can back out of the deal during the cooling off period. This usually happens if market conditions turn negative for the new issue. The other 3 answers are true.

60. C: They firm acted as a dealer; as the principal in this transaction. This is not a violation of any rules. The dealer may earn a markup on the transaction; if the dealer previously purchased this security at a lower price.

61. A: (D) describes a type of Regulation D offering. (C) is a Reg A+ offering. (B) is known as Reg S.

62. C: 2 negative GDP prints in a row is considered to be a recession.

63. D: The currency conversion rate will be determined by the EUR USD exchange rate in the spot forex currency market.

64. B: The final offering place, security delivery date and underwriter's spread must all be included in the final prospectus. The red herring is the preliminary prospectus.

65. A: A call option writer has unlimited risk.

66. A: GSEs are government sponsored entities that issue Agency Securities. Ginnie Maes are a type of agency security.

67. D: The premium paid for the long call minus the premium received for the short call equals the amount that is paid for the vertical spread.

68. C: Common stockholders do not have voting power in the matter of bankruptcy.

69. C: All qualified dividends received by ordinary income earners are taxed at a rate of 15% for the year in which they were received.

70. D: The minimum dollar amount to purchase a GNMA pass-through certificate is $1,000.

71. A: The debt service for general obligation bonds issued by the state is supported by revenue received at the state level. This revenue includes sales taxes and income taxes.

72. C: When acting as a market maker, the firm is trading for its own account and is acting as a dealer.

73. A: Buying puts will give the investor the most protection from a fall in the stock price. The investor will have set the minimum sales price for the stock as the strike price of the put.

74. A: A fund that charges a front-end load will be offered to the public at a price that is higher than its net asset value. The price known as the public offering price or POP contains the sales charge.

75. C: This is known as painting the tape, matched purchases, or matched sales.

Mock Exam 2 - Answers and Rationales

1. A - According to the Investment Company Act of 1940, financial statements are required to be sent to shareholders on a semiannual basis at the minimum.

2. B - Acting as an agent, broker-dealers normally charge commissions. Acting as principals, they markup securities sold from their own inventory.

3. A - Customers that open margin accounts must sign a hypothecation agreement to pledge their securities as collateral for loans from the broker-dealer for margin account purchases. The broker-dealer may then rehypothecate the securities to the bank, meaning that they are pledged to the bank as collateral for loans to the broker-dealer for lending to customers.

4. C - The credit quality of an exchange-traded note is based on the creditworthiness of the issuer, usually an investment bank that structures the note and sets its terms. Importantly, the credit quality is not based on the underlying portfolio for which the performance of the investment is based upon.

5. A - Cold calls can be made between 8am and 9pm in the customer's time zone. Although it is 7:30pm in California, it is actually 10:30pm in New Jersey because of the difference in time zones. Therefore, this call is prohibited.

6. D - Rights are short-term instruments that allow a shareholder to purchase the stock below its market price for a period that usually expires after 4-6 weeks. They are issued to existing shareholders in proportion to their ownership interest, so that if exercised, they allow the shareholder to maintain their percentage of ownership, or protect against dilution. Warrants are long term instruments and are often used as sweeteners in corporate bond issues. They do not protect shareholders from dilution.

7. A -Roth contributions are always made with after-tax dollars and are never tax-deductible.

8. B - Investors would now be facing reinvestment rate risk, as bonds have been called and it will be difficult to find another investment offering the same return that was available prior to the bond being called.

9. D - There are no federal dollar limits on contributions as long as they do not exceed "the amount necessary to provide for the qualified education expenses of the beneficiary." Many states do impose dollar limits on total contributions made on behalf of one beneficiary.

10. A - One of the most attractive benefits of a variable annuity is tax-deferred growth during the accumulation period. All dividends, interest, and capital gains earned during the accumulation period may be reinvested tax-free.

11. A - A firm may hold customer mail upon written request. Mail can be held for up to three months.

12. C - Closed-end company shares trade in the secondary market on exchanges. Their prices are determined by market supply and demand and therefore may be priced at a premium or discount to their NAV.

13. B - The order of liquidation in a limited partnership is secured bondholder, unsecured bondholder, limited partner, and lastly general partner.

14. C - Restricted persons include immediate family members of restricted persons. Immediate family members under this rule include spouses, siblings, children, parents, and in-laws. Grandparents, aunts, uncles, cousins, and ex-spouses are not considered restricted persons and therefore can freely invest in IPOs.

15. B - The discount rate is set by the Fed, and is the rate charged to commercial banks and other depository institutions on loans they receive from their regional Federal Reserve Bank's lending facility--the discount window. The Fed influences the Fed Funds Rate, but does not actually set the rate - it is set by the market. The prime rate is set by banks.

16. D - The healthcare industry is considered a recession-proof (i.e. defensive) sector because it remains constant regardless of the ups and downs of the economy.

17. C - A statutory disqualification occurs if the individual has been convicted a felony or a securities related misdemeanor within the past 10 years.

18. C - Under Regulation S-P, a privacy notice must be sent to a customer prior to entering into an agreement to engage in business with that client and annually thereafter.

19. B - The MSRB creates rules, but does not enforce its own rules. The MSRB rules are enforced by FINRA for securities firms. Within banks, they are enforced by the Federal Reserve, Comptroller of the Currency, and the FDIC.

20. A - Investors make after-tax contributions to 529 Plans. The earnings in the plan grow tax-free and any distributions for qualified educational expenses are tax-free at the federal level. Additionally, registered representatives must disclose that there may be certain tax benefits for opening a plan inside your state of residency, for example, tax deductions off of your state income taxes. Conversely, if an individual invests in a 529 Plan outside of their state, their state of residency might make they pay taxes on the growth of the plan.

21. C - Front-running is defined as trading on material non-public information ahead of an imminent block sale in the same or related securities

22. C - Ginnie Mae is a government agency that has the explicit backing of the US Government, while Fannie Mae and Freddie Mac have an 'implied' backing of the US government.

23. A - In a short margin account, a customer must deposit $2,000 even if the full value of the transaction is less than $2,000. This is a FINRA rule separate from the Federal Reserve Board's Regulation T.

24. C - This is the framework behind Keynesian economic theory, founded by John Maynard Keynes in the 1930's.

25. B - Preferred stock pays dividends if declared by the Board of Directors. Preferred stock generally does not have voting rights. While it has priority over common stock in the event of a corporate liquidation, it does not have priority over corporate debt, including debentures.

26. B - When an investor buys a call to protect a short stock position, the investor will breakeven when the stock price is equal to the price at which the stock was sold short minus the call premium paid. 61 – 1.50 = $59.50. The investor is bearish and will make money only when the short position can be covered at a price below this point because of the premium that was paid for the call.

27. C - The social security number of the minor is used, as the minor is the legal owner of the assets.

28. B - The Options Clearing Corporation (OCC) is the world's largest equity derivatives clearing house. As a clearinghouse, the OCC also acts as guarantor, ensuring that the obligations of the contracts it clears are fulfilled.

29. D - An investor must own stock as of the date of record in order to receive a dividend payment. To own stock by the record date, it must be purchased before the ex-dividend date which is 1 business day before the record date. By purchasing before the ex-date, there are two business days for settlement to occur, in accordance with regular way settlement process.

30. A - JoeBrokerDealer will be subject to the ban for two years after the contribution was made even if the MFP leaves the firm. JaneBrokerDealer is also subject to the ban for the same period, even though the contribution was made while the MFP was associated with another municipal securities firm.

31. D - Freeriding is the prohibited practice of entering a trade to buy securities, then selling them the following day without having had sufficient funds in the account to pay for the trade.

32. C - Total return on a bond is determined by adding the interest earned during the time period to any capital gain, then dividing this result by the initial purchase price of the bond.

33. D - A communication made available to retail investors cannot be classified as institutional. If the number of retail recipients is up to and including 25 persons, it is classified as correspondence. For larger audiences (more than 25 retail persons), it is considered retail communication.

34. C - Corporate securities are not exempt from registration under the Securities Act of 1933. They must be SEC registered.

35. D - A "breakpoint sale" is a violation that occurs when a registered rep does not disclose to the customer the opportunity to take advantage of a sales charge discount, or "breakpoint".

36. A - Industrial development bonds are issued by governments for the benefit of private corporations. Revenue streams raised by the facilities pay principal and interest. They are a form of conduit bond. Projects funded by IDRs include parking garages, factories, industrial parks, and sports stadiums.

37. D - An upward sloping, or normal yield curve, indicates that long-term interest rates are higher than short-term interest rates. This is considered normal as investors holding bonds with long-term maturities demand more interest for taking on the increased risk.

38. A - Accrued interest is measured from the last interest payment date (coupon date) up to but not including the settlement date of the trade. Settlement date is not included in these accrued interest computations because legal ownership of the bond changes on settlement date and this is the date from which the new owner of the bond begins earning his own interest.

39. D - FINRA rules prohibits broker-dealers from interpositioning a third party between the customer and broker for purposes of avoiding or evading the best execution requirement, or to generate additional fees and commissions.

40. B - Penny stocks are stocks priced below $5 per share that do not trade on an exchange. They are frequently thinly traded, which means that there may be no market for the stock if customers want to liquidate their positions. Because of this market risk additional disclosure must be made to all buyers of penny stock.

41. B - Firms must verify customer information at least once every 36 months. The point of this requirement is to ensure that the account is still appropriate and the information on file is still accurate.

42. A - Debt maturing in one year or less trades in the money market. Money market investments are attractive to investors because they offer high liquidity. Many investors access this market through money market mutual funds.

43. A - Outside business activity requires the firm to be notified of the full details of the activity. It does not, however, require permission from the firm. Borrowing money from family members does not require permission from a broker dealer.

44. C - Stock splits and reverse splits do not change the total value of investors' holdings. For example, if the investor owned 800 shares at $1 per share before the 1-for-10 reverse split, he/she will own 80 shares at about $10 per share after the event.

45. A - Because zero coupon bonds pay no interest until maturity, their prices fluctuate more than other types of bonds in the secondary market. Variable bonds have little price fluctuation because their rates adjust to current interest rates. Also, long-term bonds are generally more volatile than short-term bonds.

46. A - A bond's current yield is calculated by dividing the annual interest income by the current market price. $50/$950 = 5.26%.

47. B - Nasdaq is a negotiated market where market-makers negotiate a price with other customers and broker-dealers.

48. A - Common stock is purchased by investors for its capital appreciation potential. Historically it has kept pace with the rate of inflation and is used to meet growth objectives. It is most junior in terms of claims to assets in a corporate liquidation, and does not protect investors from investment risk.

49. B - REITs can avoid double taxation on profits passed through as dividends to shareholders by concentrating their investments in real estate. At least 75% of total assets must be in real estate, and at least 75% of gross income must be derived from real estate. Also, they must pass through at least 90% of their gains to shareholders.

50. B - A Currency Transaction Report (CTR) must be filed with FINCEN within 15 days for any cash deposits in excess of $10,000 in a single day.

51. C - Under a Tenancy in Common (or Joints Tenants in Common account), each owner has a specified percentage of the entire account. At each owner's death, his/her portion of the account is liquidated and distributed to his/her beneficiary.

52. D - QIBs generally are institutions or other entities that, in aggregate, own and invest (on a discretionary basis) at least $100 million in securities. Under Rule 144A, QIBs can freely trade private placements among themselves.

53. D - Interest income received by holders of municipal bonds is generally exempt from federal income tax and from state and local income taxes for residents of the state in which debt is issued.

54. D - When a bond is trading at a discount (market price lower than par value), the YTC will be the highest yield, then YTM, then CY, and the nominal yield the lowest yield.

55. A - ETFs are not redeemed by the issuer. Instead, investors liquidate shares by selling them on an exchange.

56. C - Short options positions have obligations that must be performed if the holder exercises the contract. Put writers have the obligation to buy stock at exercise when the put holders exercise the right to sell at the strike price.

57. A - A stock split doesn't affect the total value of stock owned. In this example, the shares are worth $9,000 before and after the split. But three times as many shares are owned. To calculate the new number of shares, multiply the shares by the first number of the split and divide by the second number of the split: 100 shares x 3 / 1 = 300 shares. Because the $9,000 is now divided among 300 shares, the new stock price will be $30 per share.

58. A - For regular way trades in equities, the ex-dividend date is one business days before the record date.

59. A - Roth IRAs are not available to everyone with earned income. Instead, only individuals who earn below a certain threshold can contribute to a Roth. In contrast, any investor with earned income is eligible to invest in a traditional IRA.

60. B - Only employee deferrals, not employer contributions, may go into the Roth account. All employer contributions go into the regular 401(k).

61. D - The SEC never approves or disapproves of securities. Instead, the SEC clears the distribution for public sale.

62. D - Unsecured bonds are also known as debentures.

63. D - SIPC coverage protects customers from financial loss in the event of the financial failure of a broker-dealer. It protects each separate customer for up to $500,000 total, but no more than $250,000 in cash. Importantly, SIPC does not protect against market losses.

64. C - The options account agreement must be signed and returned within 15 days of account approval.

65. B - An individual who is retired, or in the later stages of life, would not be likely to make an investment that could result in the complete loss of their capital, or one that would require a long-term investment horizon.

66. A - Under Regulation D, for a married couple to be accredited they must have a net worth, excluding home equity, of $1 million. The income test for married persons is a joint income of $300,000 in each of the two most recent years. This couple meets neither test.

67. C - Annuity units in variable annuity contracts fluctuate in value based on the performance of separate account assets. The number of units is fixed but their value continues to fluctuate.

68. D - Passive losses may be used to offset earnings from other passive sources only. They cannot be used to offset investment income or ordinary income.

69. B - Inflation risk is a major concern for investors who hold portfolios of fixed income investments for funding retirement income. As inflation increases, the purchasing power of their fixed coupon will fall.

70. A - The "third market" is where exchange listed securities trade in the OTC market, typically handled by a broker-dealer through its own trading system.

71. D - Under monetary policy, an increase to either the reserve requirement or the discount rate will deter lending, which will result in a tightening of the money supply. A decrease in spending by the U.S. government will also reduce the amount of money, but government spending is a tool of fiscal policy. When the Fed purchases securities in the open market more money goes into circulation, so this would ease the money supply.

72. B - A market order gives the broker instructions to buy or sell a specified quantity of securities immediately, as soon as the order reaches the market. A full execution of the order is assured but the execution price is unknown.

73. C - Investors sell their shares at the net asset value price next calculated after the order is received, which is the concept of forward pricing.

74. B - The regulatory element of continuing education must be completed on the second anniversary of initial registration, and every third year thereafter.

75. D - Confirmations must be delivered to customers at or before completion of each transaction (aka by settlement).

Mock Exam 3 - Answers and Rationales

1. A: CCO = Chief Compliance Officer.

2. C: When the term blue chip stocks is used, think of the long-establish most well-known companies that consistently perform well and have done so for a very long time. Most if not all of these are listed on the NYSE.

3. D: Occasionally, a client will be told that a trade was done at a transaction price which turns out to be incorrect. This can happen for a number of reasons, usually clerical, not intentional. Federal law and FINRA rules state clearly that the client will be told about the erroneous report, and the transaction will be done at the actual price at which it took place, not at the erroneous price. Since every transaction is a legal contract, the actual price at which the trade was executed is the legally binding price.

4. D: Exchange traded funds; Exchange traded Notes; Equity Linked Notes are all traded on the NYSE.

5. A: A customer can open a joint account with their registered rep. In that event, sharing in the performance of the account is permitted, in proportion to the contribution made by each party.

6. B: Distributions from an IRA must commence by April 1st of the year following attainment of age 70 ½.

7. C: The Office of Financial Asset Control (OFAC) maintains the list.

8. A: Once a person passes their RR exam, within 2 years from that anniversary date, a FINRA required continuing education test must be taken and passed. Then the CE tests are every three years thereafter.

9. D: Selling away is a violation. It means selling securities which are not authorized to be sold by the employing broker-dealer.

10. A: Front running is the illegal placing of an order just prior to placing a client's order so as to take advantage of the anticipated market price move.

11. D: Knowing your customer is the single most important step in the suitability of recommendations.

12. C: 8 am to 9 pm in the prospect's time zone is the law.

13. D: Monthly or quarterly, depending on whether there has been any securities activity in the account.

14. A: Government budget, spending and taxation policies are fiscal policies. Federal Reserve policies are monetary.

15. D: TIC, tenants in common, holds that each co-tenant in the account will have their % share of the account

go to their estate upon death. In joint tenancy with rights of survivorship (JTWROS), the survivor receives the share of the other co-tenant upon death.

16. B: Think of the letters S-P as Security account Privacy.

17. D: All State securities Administrators are part of the North American Securities Administrators Association (NASAA).

18. C: The federal funds rate of interest is the interbank overnight loan rate.

19. A: Slowdown in the economy implies the economy is contracting, beginning to 'shrink.'

20. D: Trades in the 3rd market are trades in stocks which are executed off the floor of the stock exchange on which those stocks are listed.

21. C: Cyclical companies tend to follow the business cycle: defensive companies tend to perform in a consistent stable way regardless of the cycle; growth companies are expected to grow faster than the economy in general.

22. D: Firm commitment implies the syndicate is purchasing the new issue from the issuer with a view to retailing it to the investing public….this is acting in a principal/dealer capacity. Best efforts underwritings are being done on an agency/brokerage basis.

23. A: Regulation D covers Private Placement offerings.

24. B: A 'weak' US dollar makes US goods 'cheaper' for foreign buyers to buy, since their currency becomes 'stronger.' This leads to an increase in the export of US manufactured goods.

25. B: What do many homeowners do when interest rates decline? They refinance their mortgage at the lower interest rate. This means the high-interest mortgages in the portfolio of the mortgage-backed product will vanish. One term used to describe the risk of this occurring is prepayment risk.

26. C: A unit investment trust typically has a fixed portfolio of securities, whereas an open end (mutual fund) makes purchases of additional securities for the portfolio on a regular and frequent basis.

27. C: Non-systematic risk is business risk --- the risk of putting all your eggs in one basket, in one company, in one business sector…..and if that business does badly, you lose. Diversification is a good way of mitigating this risk.

28. A: As described in the explanation to question #67 above, diversification is an effective way to reduce exposure to business risk.

29. A: The 529 plans are considered by the SEC and FINRA to be municipal fund securities.

30. A: Short term debt reacts the least in price when rates change.

31. B: A letter of intent is not an obligation but rather a show on one's intent to invest an amount equal or more than a mutual fund's breakpoint level so as to qualify for the reduced sales charge. LOI gives 13 months to do so.

32. B: Investment grade ratings end with the BBB rating. Below that are speculative grade ratings. BB+ would be the higher speculative rating from among these multiple-choice answers. Ba1 is a Moody's rating, not S&P.

33. A: American Depository Receipts are receipts for foreign stock and are a best way for American investors to take beneficial ownership in shares of foreign corporations.

34. C: Shorting an option contract is doing an opening sale transaction, which is writing an option contract, generating premium income.

35. D: Trades are to be reported to the appropriate 'tape' within 10 seconds of execution of the transaction.

36. B: Not only do the past unpaid dividends have to be brought current, but the current year's dividend must also be paid. Common stock cannot get any dividend payment until the cumulative preferred has been brought completely current. Therefore, a total of $5 is past due covering the shortfall in the prior 2 years, and $5 is due for the current year: $10 must be paid to get current.

37. D: An illustration is the best way to show why limited profit/limited loss is correct:

Example You purchase 100 shares of ABC stock at $50. You write/sell an ABC May 50 call for a premium of $3. If the stock falls to zero dollars per share (bankrupt), you lose $50 on the stock but get to keep the $3 premium. Net loss = $47/share. If the stock rises to infinity, your call gets exercised and you are OBLIGATED to deliver your 100 shares of ABC to the person exercising the call, and you will receive the $50 per share exercise price. You sold your stock at $50 and you had paid $50 for it initially --- you make nothing on the stock, but you get to keep the $3 premium --- your maximum gain is $3 per share. You have limited loss ($47 worst case) and you have limited gain ($3 best case).

38. B: This is the industry's definition of a 'shelf' offering – register more shares now than you intend to sell now, and save the balance for a later time, putting them 'on the shelf.'

39. C: Think of a funnel. Big institutional investors are doing many trades every day through numerous broker-dealers with which they have accounts. But all the transactions and the cash and securities clearing and settlement are 'funneled' through one firm for accounting simplicity. The prime broker is the bottom part of the funnel.

40. D: Remember the acronym D E R P --- this is the chronological order of the relevant dates when a cash dividend is declared: declaration date; ex-dividend date; record date; payable date

41. B: Failure to honor a firm quote is called 'backing away.'

42. B: Hedging investment risks involves strategies to mitigate and to reduce exposure to investment loss. Hedging is not a concept of maximizing profits.

43. C: This practice is known as 'payment for order flow' and is perfectly legal as long as the firm makes full disclosure to public customers that such an agreement exists.

44. A: The purchase needs to be paid for in a timely way or the law does not consider the purchaser to be the 'owner' of the shares and entitled to any profit on them. Regulation T refers to the use of sale proceeds to pay for the purchase as 'free-riding.' It is not acceptable.

45. A: Answer A is accurate --- short call means writing a call, which puts the investor in an obligated position to sell 100 shares of the stock at the exercise price if exercised….. assuming it's an equity option.

46. C: III and IV are two of the ways to obtain a reduced sales charge (breakpoint). Switching from one fund to another under the same sponsorship (exchange privilege) carries no sales charge at all, so a reduction is irrelevant. Reinvesting distributions is a wonderful practice, and will help reach a breakpoint, but ONLY under the ROA (rights of accumulation) program, not the 13 months LOI approach.

47. D: The regular corporation, known as the C corp., has its profits taxed under the Internal Revenue Code. The other three business types in this question are not subject to IRS taxation of their profits.

48. B: Businesses can take advantage of annual tax-deductible write-offs according to specific schedules in the internal revenue code, referred to as depreciation schedules.

49. C: Hurricanes, tornadoes, earthquakes, floods, the electric grid going down, disasters which disrupt business operations for long periods of time….. FINRA requires every brokerage firm to have a plan in place so that investors can have access to their accounts as quickly as possible ----FINRA calls it a business continuity plan.

50. D: FINRA gives a candidate three tries before imposing a six-month waiting period. Each failure from the 4th failure on requires another six-month waiting period. Once you are finished, click the button below. Any items you have not completed will be marked incorrect.

51. B: If an investor plans to reach a breakpoint within the next 13 months, he can write a letter of intent (LOI) to his broker. The LOI is a signed, nonbinding statement of the investor's intent to invest enough over the next 13 months to reach the breakpoint. In response, the broker will charge the investor the discounted sales charge on current purchases. The additional shares the customer is able to purchase due to the discount will be held aside by the mutual fund until the customer actually reaches the breakpoint.

52. C: Front-running is the practice of trading for one's own account in front of a large customer trade (for example a block trade of 10,000 or more shares), because you believe the order will impact the market price

of the security. It is a form of insider trading.

53. B: Fixed-income investors are more exposed to inflationary risk than equity investors. Thus, both Steve and Bill will be exposed to this type of risk. However, the degree of inflationary risk is higher for longer term investments. Since Steve's portfolio consists of securities that will expire within a year and Bill's does not, Bill's portfolio has more inflationary risk than Steve's.

54. D: Open market operations is when the Fed buys and sells U.S. treasury bonds on the secondary market. Open market operations (OMOs)--the purchase and sale of securities in the open market by a central bank--are a key tool used by the Federal Reserve in the implementation of monetary policy. The short-term objective for open market operations is specified by the Federal Open Market Committee (FOMC). Historically, the Federal Reserve used OMOs to adjust the supply of reserve balances so as to keep the federal funds rate--the interest rate at which depository institutions lend reserve balances to other depository institutions overnight--around the target established by the FOMC.

55. B: A defining feature of a corporation is that it offers limited liability to its investors, meaning that investors are held liable for only the amount of money they invest in the company. This means that investors' other assets are not at risk for the company's debts; nor are investors personally liable for any lawsuits that might be brought against the company. The most they can ever lose by the purchase of a company's stock is its purchase price.

56. A: The intrinsic value of an option is the difference between the strike price (40) and the market price (39) if the contract is in the money. Puts are in the money when the market price is lower than the strike price. Therefore, the intrinsic value is $1. The option was purchased for $7 and later sold for $1 (the intrinsic value), netting an overall loss of $600 (-$6 x 100).

57. A: Bonds with long maturities and low coupons have the most price volatility. Although some of the coupons are similar, maturity is the most significant factor for determining price volatility. Of the choices given, the 30 year mortgage bond has the longest time until maturity and exhibits the greatest price fluctuations when market dynamics change.

58. A: (A) is the Clearing Firm. (B) is a broker-dealer. (C) is a market maker. (D) is a transfer agent.

59. D: The FED - Federal Reserve was created in 1913 by the Federal Reserve Act to serve as the nation's central bank. These are some of the objectives of the FED.

60. C: FDIC - Federal Deposit Insurance Corporation covers up to $250,000 per depositor, per FDIC insured bank for cash held in a checking account.

61. B: To curb inflation, the FED could increase interest rates. This can reduce the rate of spending since there is less money to go around and therefore can reduce spending and slow inflation. The other 3 answers may create more inflation.

62. A: Secondary market transactions occur on stock exchanges. Dark pool transactions in large blocks are known as the fourth market while buying an IPO before the stock is listed on an exchange is the primary market.

63. C: This document that is released by the municipal security's issuer is known as the official statement.

64. D: Secured debt has priority over unsecured debt. Unsecured debt includes bonds. Lastly is the stock - with common stock being the last on the food chain.

65. C: The bond is trading below 100 (par value); so it is trading at a discount.

66. C: The registration must first be effective in order for a broker-dealer to accept payment from a customer. The other 3 are incorrect.

67. D: The S&P 500 is the broadest measure of the American economy and contains all large cap stock. Buying puts can hedge the long stock fund's risk in its portfolio.

68. A: Authorized stock is all of the answers listed, except the number of authorized shares may be changed by a vote of the shareholders.

69. A: The yield on the stock will have gone up as the price has fallen because the dividend has remained constant.

70. D: All choices listed are ways that a company can pay a dividend.

71. D: EE savings bonds are sold at a discount and at maturity are redeemed at face value, which includes the interest income.

72. D: All of the items listed must appear in the tombstone ad.

73. D: All of the choices listed are types of offerings except for Rule 149.

74. B: I is incorrect in that an option is a contract between two parties, which determines the time and price at which a security may be bought or sold.

75. C: In a custodial account, the custodian is the nominal owner of the account and carries on all transactions for the minor, the real beneficial owner of the account.

Mock Exam 4 - Answers and Rationales

1. D: In addition to maintaining control, a company may want to increase its earnings per share, fund employee stock option plans, or use shares to pay for a merger or acquisition.

2. A: The investor will receive $8 per share × 100 shares: $800 plus $1 per share because it is participating, so $800 + $100 = $900.

3. A: An ADR may represent more than one share of the company's common stock and may be exchanged for the ordinary common shares. The dividend, however, is paid in the foreign currency and is received by the investor in U.S. dollars; as a result, the investor is subject to currency risk.

4. A: An investor would expect to realize the largest gain by purchasing bonds when rates are high. The bond with the longest time left to maturity will become worth the most as interest rates fall.

5. A: A mortgage bond is secured by real estate.

6. B: The parity price is found by determining the number of shares that can be received upon conversion par / conversion price = 1,000 / 25 = 40 shares. Then the parity price equals the current market value of the convertible / no. of shares, 1,200 / 40 = $30.

7. A: When comparing a corporate bond and a municipal bond of the same quality and maturity, the corporate bond would have a higher coupon rate. Interest earned on municipal bonds is free from federal income taxes and, as such, the coupon rate is lower than equal quality corporate bonds, which are subject to taxation.

8. D: The investor purchased the Treasury bond at 95.03 or 95-3/32% of $1,000 = $950.9375

9. A: A high-quality debt instrument with less than one year to maturity, regardless of its original maturity, may trade in the money market.

10. D: The short-term maturity and the fact that the issuers have solid credit ratings make money market instruments very safe.

11. C: The discount rate is the rate that is actually controlled by the Federal Reserve Board. All of the other rates are adjusted in the marketplace by the lenders as a result of a change in the discount rate.

12. A: The Federal Reserve sets all of those except government spending.

13. D: All of the parties listed may be held liable to the purchasers of the new issue.

14. C: A company doing a rights offering will use a standby underwriting agreement whereby the underwriter will "standby" ready to purchase any shares not purchased by shareholders.

15. C: Under Rule 147, 100% of the purchasers must be in the state. The issuer must meet one of the doing-business standards as listed in the other choices.

16. B: The number of nonaccredited investors is limited to 35 in any 12-month period.

17. B: This is a very small bond issue. As such it would not make sense in many cases to pay substantial legal fees to obtain a legal opinion. These bonds are said to be ex-legal because no legal opinion was ever obtained.

18. A: Mini/maxi and best eff orts are types of underwriting commitments, not types of orders.

19. A: The order has been elected because the stock has traded through the stop price. The order has now become a limit order to sell the stock at 160.

20. B: Firms that act as market makers in Nasdaq securities are trying to make the spread, which is the difference between the bid and the ask.

21. D: The Options Clearing Corporation issues all option contracts and guarantees their performance.

22. C: The investor is long the stock and wants to protect his position. The key to the question is that he does not want to spend any additional money. In this case he must sell a call. He will receive partial protection in the amount of the premium received.

23. A: New shares will be created for the investor as soon as the mutual fund company receives the money. The investor becomes an owner of record on that day.

24. C: A 12b-1 fee is assessed by the mutual fund to cover printing of prospectuses and other promotional materials. It also covers other distribution expenses. It is an annual fee charged quarterly to the shares.

25. D: A fixed annuity does not provide protection from inflation. If inflation rises, the holder of a fixed annuity may end up worse off due to the loss of value of the dollar.

26. B: The investor may contribute to both a traditional and Roth IRA in the same year. However, the amount contributed to both accounts may not exceed the annual contribution limit.

27. A: The maximum amount that a couple may contribute to their IRAs at any one time is $22,000. Between January 1 and April 15, a contribution may be made for the prior year, the current year, or both: $5,500 × 2 × 2 = $22,000.

28. C: The money has been deposited in a Roth IRA after taxes. It is allowed to grow tax deferred. If you are over 59.5 and the money has been in the IRA for at least 5 years, then it may all be withdrawn without paying taxes on the growth.

29. C: An adult may never have a joint account with a minor.

30. B: Showing a client the past performance for a mutual fund that has only been around for 3 years is in line with the regulations. All of the other choices are violations.

31. A: Of all the investments listed, only the Ginnie Mae pass-through certificate will provide income. Ginnie Mae pass-through certificates pay monthly interest and principal payments.

32. A: The Securities Exchange Act of 1934 regulates the secondary market.

33. B: When submitting the U4 an individual is required to provide all residence information for the last 5 years. Educational background is not required. The divorce would not be reported. However, if the person changed their name as a result of the divorce, the name change would be reported.

34. D: There will be no hearing unless specifically requested by a public customer, and the decision of the arbitrator is final and binding. Claims under $50,000 will be resolved in simplified arbitration.

35. B: All of the choices listed must be included, except for the name of the principal who approved the ad for use.

36. B. The representative would have to notify her employer before working outside the office in any capacity.

37. C: The Maloney Act of 1938 was an amendment to the Securities Exchange Act of 1934 and established the NASD (now part of FINRA) as the self-regulatory organization for the over-the-counter market.

38. D: Bankers' acceptances are money market instruments and are short term; series HH government bonds can only be exchanged for mature series EE; and convertible preferred stock is a security with risk. A 90-day T-bill is considered a risk-free investment.

39. A: An investor seeking protection from interest rate risk will most likely be best suited for a portfolio of Treasury bills. As the bills mature, the investor can roll over the position into newly issued bills with new interest rates.

40. B: The investor has a large position in a thinly traded stock; as a result, the investor is subject to a large amount of liquidity risk.

41. D: A client may have a numbered account if his signature as owner is on file; broker dealers may give gifts to the employees of other broker dealers with certain restrictions. To obtain outside employment, a representative must first obtain approval from the member firm where he works.

42. D: Nonqualified accounts do not require that the owner take minimum distributions. A Roth IRA, variable annuity, and joint account do not allow owners to deduct contributions from their income. As such, the accounts are not required to take minimum distributions.

43. A: A letter of intent is good for 13 months and may be backdated by the purchaser for 3 months. The 13-

month window starts at the back date.

44. D: An investor in a mutual fund portfolio has an undivided interest in that portfolio and is not an investor or stockholder in the fund company itself.

45. C: To gain some protection and take in premium income, you would sell 100 XYZ Oct 45 calls.

46. C: The OCC or Options Clearing Corporation issues all standardized options.

47. A: An allied member may not trade on the floor. He is only allowed to call himself a member and have electronic access to the exchange.

48. C: Revenue bonds are issued through a negotiated underwriting process. The issuer will select the underwriter they would like to have offer the bonds and negotiate the terms with the underwriter directly.

49. B: An insider may sell securities under Rule 144 for 90 days.

50. B: All of the answers listed will appear in the preliminary prospectus, except the offering price and the proceeds to the company.

51. B: First you must determine the number of shares. Par / conversion price = 100 / 20 = 5, multiplied by the number of preferred shares: 5 × 100 = 500.

52. A: Each ADR represents between one to 10 shares, and ADR holders have the right to vote and receive dividends. Foreign governments put restrictions on the foreign ownership of stock from time to time.

53. C: An investor who has purchased an 8% corporate bond will receive the principal payment plus the last semiannual interest payment at maturity for a total of $1,040.

54. D: As a common stock holder, you will have the right to receive your percentage of any residual assets.

55. C: The parity price of the stock is found by using the following formulas: no. of shares = PAR / CVP, 1,000 / 20 = 50, parity price = CMV of bond / no. of shares = 1,100 / 50 = 22.

56. C: Bonds issued by a turnpike authority to improve roads would be revenue bonds and the debt service would be supported through the collection of tolls. If the collection of tolls were not sufficient to cover the bond interest, the issuing state or county may cover the shortfall out of the general revenue. Of the choices listed, the bond is the most likely to have two sources of revenue backing the payments.

57. B: T-bonds are quoted as a percentage of par to 32nds of 1%. A quote of 103.16 = 103. 16/32% × 1,000 = $1,035

58. A: The money market is a place where issuers go solely for short-term financing, typically under a year.

59. D: The two tools of the government are monetary policy, which is controlled by the Federal Reserve Board and controls the money supply, and fiscal policy, which is determined by the president and Congress and controls government spending and taxation.

60. D: Purchasers of stock that has just gone public must get a prospectus for 25 days if the stock is Nasdaq listed.

61. C: Rule 145 covers mergers involving a stock swap or offer of another company's securities in exchange for its current stock.

62. C: General obligation bonds will be advertised in the daily bond buyer and the official notice of sale will provide details on the bidding procedure.

63. B: Selling stock short will expose an investor to unlimited risk because there is no limit as to how high a stock price can go.

64. B: Call sellers and put buyers are both bearish. They want the value of the stock to fall.

65. (c) A mutual fund calling itself a diversified fund is limited to owning no more than 10% of any one company.

66. C: A 12B-1 fee may be up to ¼ of 1% of the NAV.

67. B: The retirement account is qualified, which means the investor has deposited the money pretax, therefore, all of the money is taxed when it is withdrawn.

68. C: The rule is one custodian and one minor for each UGMA account. There is not a rule regarding who must be custodian.

69. A: This is a violation known as trading ahead.

70. D: Using the pending dividend to create an urgency on the part of the investor to purchase this stock is a perfect example of this violation, and the results are listed in the first three answers.

71. B: A member firm may charge a customer a larger than ordinary commission for the execution of a specific order so long as it is disclosed to the customer. A member firm must always execute a customer's order.

72. D: The part-time sales assistant who takes orders from customers must be registered because she is taking orders.

73. A: Generic advertising may not contain information about past recommendations.

74. C: The Uniform Practice Code regulates the way members conduct business with other members.

75. C: If an investor may lose part or all of his capital, it is called capital risk.

CPSIA information can be obtained
at www.ICGtesting.com
Printed in the USA
LVHW060250290422
717548LV00009B/163